# MANNY'S LAW
## The Death of Our Son

REYNALDO PRIETO

Copyright © 2018 Reynaldo Prieto
All rights reserved
First Edition

PAGE PUBLISHING, INC.
New York, NY

First originally published by Page Publishing, Inc. 2018

ISBN 978-1-64214-054-5 (Paperback)
ISBN 978-1-64214-055-2 (Digital)

Printed in the United States of America

# Preface

Twelve years ago, my son needlessly died. He was the victim of a system that we have in this great country. I'm talking about our "for profit" health-care system we have here in the USA. This form of health care failed my eldest son. He unfortunately got a serious illness and was denied care because of the lack of insurance. He became victim to a situation beyond his control. He had no insurance because he changed jobs, where he had insurance to another job where his insurance came too late to help him. Then once he got insurance, he fell victim to the preexisting condition. This, I believe, should not happen here in this great country of ours.

My wife and I, with the help of local politicians, got a law passed in New York State. This law is known as Manny's Law. We wanted to make sure he did not die in vain. My wife and I took all our pain, anguish, and grief and channeled all that emotion, and with the grace of God, it was accomplished. We were determined to prevent this horror to happen to anyone again. We were determined to stop the business as usual that exists in this flawed system.

We tried to educate our fellow New Yorkers about this new law. Unfortunately, we are just two people and our efforts are limited. Although we know firsthand that Manny's law has saved lives, we feel that most New Yorkers don't know about this law. So I decided to write this book—to tell the story not only in New York but to the entire nation, perhaps even the world. This story is a black eye to the nation.

After you read this book, I pray that we as Americans change this system. We need universal health care in America. Then as I was writing and investigating statistics about our system as compared to rest of the world, I was shocked at the statistics. That made me more determined to inform my fellow Americans to these facts. I hope that these statistics spark and energize us into action, to change a flawed system into a system we can all live with.

Manny's story is just one of many. To all the other families and victims of the way things are in this great country of ours, I write this story for you also. As a fellow victim, I stand in solidarity with you. I truly send you all my condolences as one who has suffered the same sense of loss. I feel your pain as one who has felt that pain. What they did to our loved ones is criminal, and it should have been treated as such.

In this book I compare the way Manny was treated with how my younger son was treated when he too got sick. My younger son had health insurance. Although he got his treatment, I wanted to show the flaws in the system. I pray that this will be an eye-opener to all!

THIS IS THE story of our twenty-four-year-old son; his name was Manuel Nickie Lanza Jr., a young man that was proud to be an American. He was an individual that was full of life and lived it with joy and vigor. He never dwelled on the bad but always found the good in people and in life itself. He was a hardworking and kind-hearted individual. He was an inspiration not only to his family but also to his peers. Unfortunately, his life was cut short because of the greed of his doctors and hospitals that didn't care for him and left him to die.

You might think that this couldn't happen here in America. Actually, that's what I thought also, but yes, this did happen here in the great USA, the richest country in the world. Manny was left to die because he had no health insurance. This was because he changed jobs where he had insurance to a new job and had to wait to get to full-time status to get new insurance. He was neglected and did not receive the care that he needed. The delays in his health care brought about his demise. This resulted in the worst horror that any parent can go through, having to watch their child die and then having to bury him.

Before I start my story, however, I would like to tell you about the physician's oath. This is an oath that all physicians take when they become doctors. It is called the declaration of Geneva, and as currently published by the World Medical Association, it reads as follows:

> I solemnly swear to consecrate my life to the service of humanity. I will give to my teachers the

respect and gratitude that is their due. I will practice my profession with conscience and dignity. The health of my patient will be my number one consideration. I will respect the secrets that are confided in me, even after my patient has died. I will maintain by all the means in my power the honor and the noble traditions of the medical profession. My colleagues will be my sisters and brothers. I will not permit consideration of age, disease or disability, creed, ethnic origin, gender, race, political affiliation, nationality, sexual orientation, social standing, or any other factor to intervene between my duty and my patient. I will maintain the ultimate respect for human life. I will not use my medical knowledge to violate human rights and civil liberties, even under threat; I make these promises solemnly, freely, and upon my honor.

As you will see, his doctors broke this oath.

This all started on September 17, 2004. That's the day the phone rang at about 4:00 a.m., and my wife and I were awakened out of a sound sleep. I just knew that this couldn't be good news. I answered the phone that was on the night table by my side of the bed. It was Manny telling me that he was in the hospital. He was taken to Brookhaven Hospital, which is our local hospital. He wanted me to go pick him up. I asked him what had happened, and he told me he passed out and he was taken by ambulance to the hospital. Then I told him that I was on my way.

I got up got dressed and rushed to the emergency room. My wife stayed at home because my younger son was sleeping, and we didn't want to leave him alone. We both thought that I was just going to go and pick him up and bring him home. How wrong we were. I arrived at his bedside, and there he was, lying in the bed with the hospital gown that is given to all patients while they are in the hospital. He gave me a smile and said hi. I asked him if he was okay. Again he smiled and answered yes. Again I asked him what had happened to him. He told me, "I passed out."

Then he went into detail. He told me that he got out of work and his friends were driving him home. They stopped for gas, and he just passed out, he said. The next thing he remembered was waking up here in the hospital. I asked him why he had passed out. "Were you using any cleaning solvents at work?"

He answered, "No, I don't know why I passed out."

I asked him if the doctor had told him anything.

He told me, "No, I haven't been told a thing."

So we sat there chatting about different things. I was trying to figure out in my mind what might have caused him to pass out.

Finally the emergency room doctor entered, and he identified himself to me. He asked me who I was and asked Manny if it was okay to talk about his condition with me present. Manny said, "Of course, he's my dad."

Then I asked the doctor, "What caused Manny to pass out?"

He said he ordered an X-ray and a CAT scan, which were already done. Then I got the news. Manny had arteriovenous malformation, or AVM. The doctor asked us if we knew what that was. Manny didn't, but I did. "Yes," I answered. "I have a friend that has that condition."

But since Manny didn't know, the doctor explained. He said that this was a tangle of abnormal blood vessels connecting arteries and veins in the brain. He went on, saying, "The arteries bring oxygen-rich blood to the brain, and the veins bring oxygen-depleted blood back to the lungs and heart. The AVM interferes with this process." He also warned of possible rupture of the AVM causing bleeding, which can cause a stroke, paralysis, or even death. He said it was severe and that he ordered an MRI and that Manny was going to be admitted to be evaluated by neurology, to see about the correct treatment for his condition. The doctor then asked if we had any questions. We didn't and he left.

Manny looked like he was in shock. I tried to reassure him, telling him about my friend who had the same condition. "He was treated, and he is alive and living a normal life." This kind of made him feel better. But I saw the fear in his eyes. I told him, "I'm going home to get your mom, and we would right back."

"Okay," he said. "I'll see you later."

On the way home, I was trying to figure out how I was going to tell my wife. I really wasn't looking forward for the task, but I had no choice. While I was driving, I kept going over and over different ways I was going to tell her. I must have gone over a dozen different versions of how I was going to break the news.

When I got home, my wife, Levia, was cleaning up. She had woken up my younger son and got him off to school. She asked me where Manny was. "I thought he was coming home with you."

"I thought so too, but they want to admit him." I saw her go into a panic.

"Why?" she asked.

I told her in detail all that had happened. I told her he had an AVM. She knew what that was, and her face said it all. It was a combination of fear, concern, and dread. She absorbed the information, and I knew she was crying inside. I told her to get ready; we had to go back to the hospital. She dropped everything and got dressed.

We went back to the hospital and back to Manny's bedside. Again Manny gave us his wonderful smile, and Levia gave him a hug and a kiss. She asked him how he felt. He said he felt fine. He actually looked good.

A short time later, he was taken by radiology to get his MRI done. When they brought him back, he was asleep. It turned out he didn't get his MRI done. He had suffered another seizure while he was in radiology. Then Levia leaned over him and kissed him, and I heard her say to him in a way only a mother can say, "I love you, and you better not leave me. I don't want to live life without you," with tear-filled eyes.

A short time later, he was officially admitted into the intensive care unit (ICU) of the hospital.

Now came the time where we had to make phone calls, first my job to tell them I wouldn't be in, then to my parents, who didn't take the news well. They told me they were on their way. I told my sister who also didn't take the news well and also said she was on her way.

Then Levia called her sister who lived close by, and she came to the hospital. Then she called the rest of her family, most of whom live in Pennsylvania. They all expressed their sympathy, and all said they would pray for Manny.

My family and Levia's sister arrived, and since only two visitors were allowed at a time, they visited with him in pairs. We all spent the rest of the day visiting with him and chatting among ourselves, all wondering what was to come.

Manny finally went for his MRI. He went through numerous tests, including blood tests, and was given an antiseizure medicine called Dilantin. I had to take Levia back home because my younger son would be getting home from school. So we left and returned home. When my younger son returned from school, we told him what had happened and asked him if he wanted to see his brother. He said no, he didn't want to see Manny in a hospital bed. He said, "Tell him I love him, and I hope he feels better real soon."

Since he was fourteen years old, we knew that he was capable of being home alone. We fed him and left him doing homework and returned to the hospital. We stayed with Manny for the rest of the day, and when visiting hours were over, we said our good-byes and went home.

On the way home, I expressed my concerns to Levia about the fact that Manny had no health insurance. She said, "So what? We live in America. They have to take care of him." She said, "They bring people into this country from other countries to treat them for their illnesses. Why won't they take care of Manny?"

I agreed with her and told her, "You're right."

Little did we know how wrong we were. Lack of health insurance was a problem, and we were about to find out.

The next day was a Saturday, and since I'm off on the weekends, I didn't have to worry about work. We all woke up, and my wife made breakfast for all. We ate and got ready for another day at the hospital. Again we asked my younger son if he wanted to see his brother, and he again declined. He just didn't want to see his brother in a hospital bed. You could see by his expression that he was worried about his older brother. So my wife prepared a lunch for him. We got dressed and went back to Brookhaven.

When we arrived at Manny's bedside, he told us, "I'm going home today."

We were surprised. Yesterday we were told that that Manny's condition was serious. Now he was telling us he was going home. My wife and I went to the nurse and asked her if he was really going home.

She said, "Yes, the doctors were going to discharge him today."

I said, "I thought his condition was serious." She didn't answer, then I said, "Are you are going to discharge him right out of ICU? No downgrade first?"

She said that wasn't unusual.

I answered, "Really! I worked for Mid Island Hospital as a pharmacy technician, and I know that a person is in fact not discharged out of ICU, not without a downgrade to a regular room first." I also said, "The only way a person is discharged out of an intensive care unit is either a transfer to another hospital or to the morgue because they are dead. This doesn't have anything to do with the fact that he doesn't have health insurance?"

Her face turned pale, and she said, "No, of course not."

As it turns out, this was the reason.

I left the intensive care unit and called my sister, who was a clinical pharmacist. I told her, "They are going to release Manny from the hospital right out of ICU."

She also said, "What? Without a downgrade? That's not right." I told her what the nurse said, and my sister said, "Aren't they afraid of hemorrhaging?"

"Apparently not," I answered.

"I'm coming to the hospital," she said. "I'll see you soon."

With that I returned to his bedside. The nurse was frantically trying to get a hold of the neurologist who was going to discharge Manny. She finally did, and I was told that he wanted to talk to me. He identified himself and told me that Manny was going to be discharged. I told him what I had told the nurse. He seemed to get hot under the collar.

He said, "Listen, we just don't have the facility to treat your son's condition."

"Really?" I answered. "This is a trauma hospital with a neurology department. How can you not have the facility to treat his condition?"

"Well, we don't, so I am discharging him."

"Aren't you afraid of hemorrhaging?"

This caught him off guard, and he said, "Look, we know what we are doing. You are just giving into unjustified fear. It is better to treat him as an outpatient by another neurologist."

"Really?" I said. "You know what you are doing, huh? I'm telling you right now that if anything happens to my son, I will hold you personally responsible, and I will sue you for all your worth."

Now he was really annoyed and said, "Put the nurse back on the phone."

I gave the phone to the nurse, and I said to her loud enough for him to hear, "The jerk wants to talk to you."

She got on the phone, and although I couldn't hear what he said, I could tell that he was irate, and he barked new orders to the nurse, who looked mortified.

A short time later, my sister came in and walked over to the bedside. I told her the conversation I had with the doctor. Then she went to the nurses' station, identified herself, and told her she was a clinical pharmacist and expressed her concerns. The nurse realized that we weren't going to accept the early discharge, not without a fight. By this time, Levia's sister entered the ICU department, and since there were three people at the bedside and she was a member of the NYPD, she flashed her badge and she was permitted to stay. By this time, the nurse looked nervous. First the parents, then a pharmacist, and now a cop. The nurse said she would call the doctor again.

Now we were told that he wouldn't be discharged. But now the hospital was frantically looking for a place to "dump" Manny. We as a family stayed by Manny's bedside in solidarity. A short time later, we were told by the nurse that they were making arrangements to transfer him to St. Luke's Roosevelt Hospital located in Manhattan. Then a short time later, a woman from social service came in to start an application for Manny to get Medicaid. We went through the application process, then we were told that if we were asked about insurance, to say he was Medicaid pending. I had a sense of relief, and so did my wife. We thought for sure he would now be taken care of. Again how wrong we were.

A short time later, we were told that Manny would not be going to St. Luke's Roosevelt Hospital, that they didn't have a bed for him. Later we found out after we obtained Manny's records that it was noted in his records, and I quote, "Received call from St Luke's Hospital. Pt will not be going there today because: first pt is Medicaid pending and they have an issue with that . . ." This was signed by the nurse, dated and time stamped. Also another sheet, which was the patient's assessment report, stated, and I quote, "Patient's need for services may be restricted due to lack of insurance." This shows that insurance was an issue as to why my son did not get proper care. So Manny stayed in Brookhaven for another night.

The next day, Sunday, the third day at Brookhaven, we went back to the hospital, and Manny was still in intensive care. Now we were told that Manny was being transferred to St. Luke's Roosevelt Hospital. We were also told that they were having trouble finding an ambulance, and since they were a privately owned and operated company and since Manny did not have insurance, they wanted payment in advance. So much for the private sector providing better care, as we are told by our politicians. We were again angry and expressed our concerns. We offered to pay for the ambulance. Finally, after much fanfare, the patient advocate got him an ambulance. My wife, Manny, and all his records and an order to have an angiogram done were put in the ambulance, and off they went to St. Luke's Roosevelt Hospital located on West 59 Street in Manhattan. My wife later told me that she was reassuring Manny, telling him that she loved him and that he would be fine.

I, however, had to go home to attend to my younger son. I fed him and saw to his needs. Then off I went to the long ride to St Luke's. My mother took the ride with me, and it took about two hours to arrive. When we arrived, Manny was already admitted. He was put under the care of Dr. Yashuniri Niimi and Dr. Alejandro Berenstein, whom, at this time, we hadn't even met yet. My mother and I went to his room, and he was already settled in. Not much was done that day except routine blood work, medication and blood pressure, temperature, etc., but the angiogram wasn't done yet. We stayed the rest of day with him, and when visiting hours were over, we said our good-byes and left. We all had the feeling that a part of us was left behind. And so ended his first day at St. Luke's Hospital.

The ride home, as you can imagine, was one full of emotions. We were concerned about the outcome of his treatment. With tear-filled eyes, we talked about our son, who was facing a life-threatening condition, and how he was being ignored. We fought back the tears, and with every conversation, the words kept getting stuck in our throats because we couldn't talk without crying. We were in disbelief. How could this have happened? Manny was always so healthy. There was no sign until now that he was even sick. After all, a seizure is a sign that something is wrong. We silently said our prayers and hoped for the best. When we arrived home, we tried, for our younger son's sake, to keep some normalcy in our lives.

The next day was Monday; it was Manny's second day at St. Luke's. We left my younger son home from school because we didn't know how long we were going to be in Manhattan. We fed him breakfast and my wife made lunch, and we left for Manhattan. When we arrived at the hospital, Manny was in his room, watching TV. We asked him if he had the angiogram done. He told us that he hadn't but that a team of doctors came to see him. Again nothing but routine stuff was done and no new information. We asked when they were going to do the angiogram, and we were told it was pending. We stayed with him till about 5:00 p.m., and we left.

The next day, Tuesday, day 3 at St. Luke's, the angiogram still wasn't done. My wife was upset and asked to speak with his doctors. We were told that his doctors were making rounds and that they would come in and talk to us shortly. After about an hour and a half, my wife again asked when the doctors were coming to see us, and she was told, "They'll get to you when they get to you." My wife kept her composure for Manny's sake. Anyway, *shortly* meant about three hours later. Finally Manny's doctors, Dr. Yashuniri Niimi and Dr. Alejandro Berenstein, who, by the way, didn't identify themselves and who were supposed to be the top specialist to treat Manny for his condition, arrived. Dr. Berenstein arrogantly told us that "Manny's condition required a special angiogram machine that we are getting in three weeks. This way we could evaluate correctly his condition and give the proper treatment." He was scheduled for November 11, 2004, for a follow-up. We were given a script for Dilantin and were sent on our way. It felt like "Don't let the door hit you in the butt on the way out." They didn't even escort him out. We borrowed a wheelchair from the floor, and we took him out ourselves. I went to get the car, and we left the wheelchair in the lobby and went home.

Levia got a card and wrote Manny a note in the card. She wanted to reassure him and show him her love. This is what was written on the back of the envelope:

P.S.
All I can say is I wish it was me **not you**.

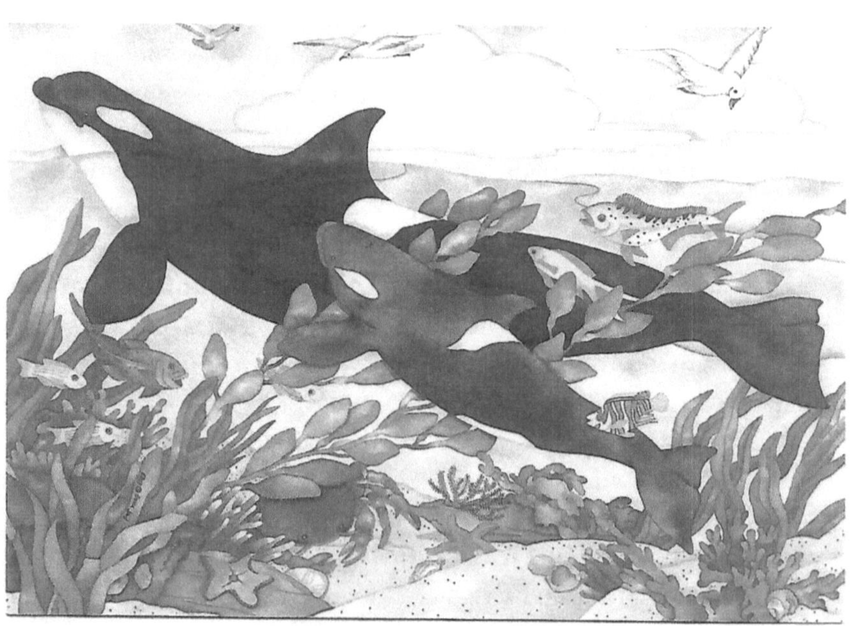

This was the front of the card

This was on the inside of the card:

9-21-04

Dear and wonderful Son of Mine!

Sometimes things happen in life so you can **STOP** and smell the flowers. I know that you are a **strong person** and that so many people love you and are praying for you, in time you **will** be **walking** everywhere, and doing all the things that you love. So don't worry, about your JOB right now only your health and getting better. Manny you are in the best of care with the tops of Doctor's helping you. God gives you as much as you can handle. Just let us take one day at a time. And when you know it you will be home with us, where you belong. I love you **always** so don't you ever forget and if you need anything let me know. See you soon. I need you home I feel lost without you, part of me is missing. Now I know you are the best part of me. I love you son!
Mom

Now I know how we felt as parents about this whole ordeal. Can you imagine what Manny, "the patient," felt about this? How worried he must have felt not only because he had a life-threatening condition but also of how we were now fighting for him to get the proper care that he so desperately needed. How he must have silently suffered, knowing that money meant more than his life. This is something that no one should have to face. He never smoked, he never drank alcohol, he took care of himself physically, and most of all, he never had a serious illness. He was proud to be an American, and this was his thanks.

When we got home, Manny he went to his room. My wife attended to the boys, and I left to fill his prescription at the local pharmacy, only to find out that he was given a twenty-day supply and his follow-up was scheduled for November 11, seven weeks later. We didn't have enough Dilantin. I paid for the medicine and left. When I got home, I told my wife that he wasn't given enough medicine. So she called the doctor's office. She got a hold of the clinical coordinator. Now in our opinion, this woman was the most unprofessional, uncaring, callous health-care professional we have ever had the misfortune to deal with. Levia told her about the medicine situation, and she was told, "Oh, no, you have to see a physician in your area if you want more medicine."

Levia asked, "Why does he need to see another physician when you guys are the doctors that are taking care of him?"

She simply refused to call in another script. She told my wife, "My kids have insurance. Why doesn't your son have any?"

I'll never forget the look of anguish in Levia's face.

My wife tried repeatedly calling the doctor's office, desperately trying to get more medicine and constantly being told by the coordinator, "You need to obtain insurance if you want him to be taken care of."

Day by day she pleaded with this uncaring person. I really don't know what the big deal was to call the pharmacy so that my son could get more medicine. When Manny was down to his last days of medicine, she didn't know what to do. Finally, in desperation, she called the patient advocate at Brookhaven Hospital. She told my wife, "There has to be a clinic in your area, take him there." So my wife got the number of the health-care clinic and made an appointment so my son could see a doctor.

The appointment was made that same day. Unfortunately, my wife doesn't drive and I was at work in Manhattan, and no neighbors were available. So Manny and she walked about two miles to go see a doctor. There he was seen by Dr. Sabrina Johnson. I would like at this time to say this woman was a blessing. She knew that Manny had no insurance, but that didn't matter to her. Manny was her only concern. She saw him, monitored his Dilantin levels, and was the only doctor that attended to Manny. She just couldn't understand what the delay was about. She was a compassionate person. May God bless her always. She gave him more Dilantin, so at least he had his medicine.

My wife called the coordinator daily to try to schedule his angiogram, and every day she was told Manny needed to get insurance. My wife said he was Medicaid pending. The coordinator kept saying, "That's not good enough. When you obtain insurance, we'll take care of him."

So started the race to get Manny the care he needed. Little did we know it was a race to save his life, a race that unfortunately we lost, and Manny paid the ultimate price.

So my son again went to see Dr. Johnson at the clinic for his follow-up. My wife explained to her the difficulty she was having trying to schedule his angiogram. The doctor said, "What are they waiting for? He needs to be treated." The doctor called Stony Brook Hospital, a state hospital that was relatively close. She explained the situation, and she gave my wife a referral to have Manny evaluated for treatment. But as fate would have it, when my wife got home, there was a message on the answering machine, setting Manny's angiogram for November 4, 2004. She called Dr. Johnson and told her they scheduled Manny for November 4. She asked her, "Should I go to Stony Brook, or should I take him to St Luke's?"

Dr. Johnson said, "Take him to St. Luke's. Let them finish what they started. They are the top in the field of neurology."

So Levia confirmed his appointment, and so he was set to have his angiogram done.

The day came for Manny to have his angiogram done. We drove into Manhattan to St. Luke's Roosevelt Hospital. We went to the floor where we were told to go and check Manny in. They prepped Manny, and they took him to have it done. A while later, we were told that it was over and that someone would come and talk to us soon. A short time later, a health-care professional came in and told us that Manny needed to have his procedure done "like yesterday." She asked us if we knew what was to be done to Manny. We told her that no one had explained anything. So she got into detail explaining everything. She even drew pictures to show us the procedure.

An embolization has been used to treat AVMs since the early 1980s. This procedure involves the injection of glue or other nonreactive liquid adhesive material into the AVM in order to block it off. For this purpose, a small catheter or tube is passed through a groin vessel all the way up into the blood vessels in the head supplying the AVM. This is why angiogram was done. An angiogram is a road map of sorts that show the path of blood vessels throughout the body. With this road map, they can see which is the best route to take the catheter into the head.

We were told that Manny's condition was severe, that he had numerous AVMs, and that he needed to have numerous procedures to possibly correct them. She went on to tell us that Manny had large blood vessels called arteries pumping blood into small blood vessels called veins. She said that normally, capillaries, which are fine blood vessels and reduce the blood flow which reduces the pressure of the blood entering the veins. This process prevents the veins from rupturing. Then she explained it in layman's terms so we could understand it better. She explained capillaries are like a faucet or valve that reduces the higher pressure from the arteries to lower pressure to the veins. Then she said Manny didn't have any capillaries and that the arteries were pumping blood directly to his veins. They wanted to place an embolism or a restriction between the arteries and veins to reduce the blood flow. She told us that the first of several procedures was to be done on November 11, 2004, which was a week from that day.

My wife and I thought this person was either a physician or a physician assistant due to the extent of knowledge that she had in Manny's condition. Unfortunately, we didn't get her name or her title. This was something that we regret not doing. She did identify herself, but unfortunately, we don't remember her name or title. We were so stunned, because this was the first time that we were told what was going to be done to Manny and just how severe it was. No one up to this point said anything to us about his condition or his treatment, not his doctors or anyone else that had treated Manny.

Again Manny was discharged from the hospital, and again he wasn't escorted out. We again borrowed a wheelchair that was nearby, and we escorted our son out of the hospital. This time he was groggy from the anesthesia he had received before his angiogram. I went and got the car while they waited in the lobby. We got Manny in the car, and again we left the wheelchair in the lobby and went home. It was kind of silent ride home; we were all contemplating what was to come.

After we got home and Manny was getting over his anesthesia, we went to go talk to him. He told us he was willing to do the emobilizations, but he told us he did not want them to open his skull. He didn't want to go through that kind of operation. He didn't want to become a vegetable. We promised him, since we were his health-care proxies, that we wouldn't allow that. We spent the rest of the week living our lives as normally as possible. But we always had that nagging feeling of the risks involved in the procedure he was to have. We always thought positive, but the thought of the risks always lingered.

So Manny was to have his first embolization the morning of November 11, 2004. The evening before, my cell phone rang. I saw that it was an area code 212 number. That is a Manhattan number. I thought that it was a call to confirm Manny's procedure. I answered the phone and said hello. They caller said that this was Dr. Niimi's office and asked if this was Manny. I told them that I was his father and that I also was one of his health-care proxies and told them they could speak to me. The person said, "We are calling to cancel Manny's procedure. Dr. Niimi had an emergency and had to go Japan."

"What? How can this be? Isn't there anyone else that can cover for him?" I was told that they didn't have this information, and then I asked, "When will my son have his procedure done?" I was told that we had to call the office and reschedule. "Okay, thanks for calling," and I hung up the phone.

I was close to home; I was driving home from work. I arrived home, and my wife was coming out of a neighbor's house where she was having tea. I told my wife that I had just gotten a call from the hospital and they cancelled Manny's procedure.

"What? How can they do that?" she said.

I told her, "Dr. Niimi had an emergency and had to go to Japan."

Then she said, "Is that the only surgeon there?"

I said that they didn't have that information and that she had to call the office to reschedule.

Then she said something that as long as I live I will never forget. She said, with tears flowing from her eyes, "They are going to let Manny die. Oh my god, they are going to let him die."

We went to the phone, and we saw that they had called the house first, but obviously they didn't want to leave a message. My wife called the doctor's office and put the phone on speaker, and again she had to deal with the coordinator. My wife asked her why they had to cancel Manny's procedure. She again said to my wife that Dr. Niimi had an emergency and had to go to Japan. My wife asked, "Isn't there anyone else that can do the procedure besides Dr. Niimi?"

The coordinator answered, "No, and by the way, has Manny gotten his Medicaid yet?"

Everything kept going back to insurance.

"No, not yet. I haven't heard anything yet." They went back and forth about insurance. My wife lost her composure and told Mary, "Tell one of those assholes [Dr. Niimi or Dr. Berenstein] to call me immediately." The coordinator hung up the phone abruptly. Now my wife is a very easygoing, well-spoken person. She never talks like that. You have to understand, she lost her patience by this point.

A couple of hours or so later, the phone rang. The caller ID showed that it was the doctor's office. My wife immediately answered the phone and put the phone on speaker. The caller, who was a male, never identified himself and asked very rudely if this was Manny's mother. My wife answered yes, it was. He said to her, "Why are you trying to rush your son under the knife?"

My wife expressed her concerns about Manny's care. He answered, "We know what we are doing."

My wife said, "Listen, I'll sell my house. Please take care of Manny. Death is final." Then my wife complained about the coordinator, and he seemed annoyed about that. She continued, "I just want to schedule him for his procedure, and all I hear from her is, 'Did you get insurance? My children have insurance. Why doesn't yours?'" He then interrupted Levia and told her to call someone else in the office, that my wife was annoying her.

Imagine that, my wife was upsetting her. What about my wife, and more importantly, what about Manny? Then he gave my wife the name of the other woman who, by the way, my wife never spoke to. She only ever dealt with the very unprofessional coordinator. Then he hung up the phone. Now this person never identified himself like I said. He did, however, have a very thick accent, not a Japanese accent, more like a Latin accent. We assume it was Dr. Alejandro Berenstein, who is Spanish, and he seemed very full of himself, very arrogant.

My wife spent the greater part of her time every day after that trying to reschedule Manny's procedure. Every day my wife kept hearing about insurance: "He needs to get insurance." "When you obtain insurance, we'll take care of him." "Did you get his Medicaid yet," and so on. It got to be quite pathetic. My wife again told the coordinator what she told the doctor. "Listen, I'll sell my house. Please just take care of my son. Death is final. Do you understand?"

I guess that wasn't good enough, because the insurance game didn't seem to end. May God have mercy on her soul.

Then I told my wife, "Hey, let's get Senator Trunzo involved. He was our local state senator, and we got his number from a letter we got in the mail. My wife called his office and told them of our situation. They said they would help. We were optimistic that they would. About two days later, we got a call from Kevin Casey, a case worker from social service who was instructed from Senator Trunzo's office to expedite Manny's application. My wife called him and was asked for several papers, including pay stubs, proof of rent, and countless other papers that seemed like an endless barrage of paperwork. So now we thought Manny would get his Medicaid. Turns out we were wrong again.

Trying to deal with social service is a nightmare, let me tell you. I can't tell you how many times I saw my wife on the phone, trying to get Medicaid for Manny. They always put her on hold, and she would patiently wait to try to get Manny help. She would wait hours upon hours day after day, spending her day with the phone in her hand and tears in her eyes, trying desperately to talk to Kevin Casey; he was no help at all. Many times while she was on hold for an hour or so, they would just hang up on her, and she would immediately call them back, only to be placed on hold again. When she did finally talk to him on rare occasions, he would ask for more papers, whether it be proof of income or some other proof of something. Much of it were papers we had already sent them. We sent them whatever he asked for over and over, whether we had already sent it or not. She just wanted to get help for our son. All those hours she spent on the phone turned out to be a complete waste of time.

So my wife spent her days of the week with her endless calls to the doctor's office and social service. She even called the patient advocates at St. Luke's Hospital for advice and guidance. She spent her days waiting for hours on hold, literally being ignored. She spent her time calling and waiting during the daytime hours and crying at night. She did everything a mother can do to try to save her son's life. Every possible avenue of help turned out to be a brick wall. She was racing to get Manny his care and, as it turned out, to save his life.

Then on December 2, 2004, we got a call from the doctor's office; they scheduled Manny for February 11, 2005, for his first treatment. My wife and I were concerned about the length of time we had to wait. She asked if there was any possible way to make it sooner. They said no and they would send info in the mail concerning his pre-op instructions as well as time and date of where he needed to report. I'm sure that they figured that his Medicaid would be in place by this time.

We spent Christmas with our family, and I made sure that Manny as well as my younger son got everything they wanted for Christmas. We had a wonderful day exchanging gifts and just enjoying time with the family. Christmas dinner was to be at my parents' house. Manny got to spend what was to be his last time with his cousins, and he was the life of the party. We all had a wonderful time. But always in the back of our minds was the fact that he was facing a life-threatening condition, and no one seemed to care about it except his family.

We spent the days leading up to the New Year as a family, just enjoying being together. I would play video games with the kids, trying to make life as normal as possible. This, I can assure you, was a lot easier said than done. But we did the best we could, and life kind of felt normal. Manny as usual was his cheerful self, spending time with his brother. We watched movies as a family, and considering the circumstances, we had fun. I can't tell you how many times I cried in private, not letting anyone know that I was dying inside. I was the man of the house and had to stay or appear strong for my family's sake.

Then on December 31, 2004, we got a letter from social services stating that Manny had been denied his Medicaid. It stated, "See copy of budgets." It turned out that ten thousand dollars was too much money to earn in one year. To add insult to injury on his denial, it also stated that he wasn't eligible for Family Health Plus. So here it was. Manny was not eligible for assistance. Happy New Year, I thought. Manny never complained about anything during this ordeal. However, my wife asked him what he thought about this situation. Manny responded, "I can't understand why they won't take care of me." To this we had no answer except "greed."

We spent a quiet New Year's Eve at home, and we celebrated the New Year with enthusiasm, looking forward for the New Year and the prospects it would bring. We spent the day playing video games, eating, and just being together as a family. Then at midnight, we wished each other a happy New Year, especially to Manny, whom we thought was going to finally get his care and get better, to live a long and happy life for many years to come. Now Manny was a Star Wars fan, and he kept counting the days for the final installment of the movies, *Star Wars III: Revenge of the Sith*. He kept saying, "I can't die yet. I have to see this movie to see how the saga ends." Now in retrospect, it was like he knew his days were numbered. Unfortunately, he never got to see this movie in life.

The day after New Year's, Levia called social service to ask why Manny was denied assistance. She was told that he made too much money. Can you imagine $10,000 being too much money? Levia then asked what could be done to get him approved. We were told that he could ask for a fair hearing to protest the decision. So of course we went through the process of asking for a fair hearing. This was granted for a later date. But of course, this was to be too late to help Manny.

Then January 6, 2005, came. I remember it like it was yesterday. I came home from work early because it was a light day and I finished my scheduled workload. Manny wasn't feeling well that day. My wife and I asked him if he had a headache, which was a symptom of his condition. He answered us and said no. He was in his room, and he was just lying in his bed and said his stomach was bothering him. After a short time, Manny went to the bathroom, and when he came out, he said, "Ma, I just threw up."

We again asked him, "Does your head hurt, or are you dizzy?" He said no. So we didn't think much else of the severity of it. We thought he just had a bellyache. When dinnertime came, we decided to get food from Wendy's, which ironically was where he had worked. Levia asked Manny if he wanted anything. He said to get him a cheeseburger and french fries. We told our younger son to keep an eye on Manny, and he, being the wise guy he is, said, "I will, but only if you bring me a Checker's milkshake." I agreed.

My wife and I went to Blockbuster to get a video. We went to Wendy's to get the food. Finally we went to Checker's to get the milkshake, then we went home. My wife gave Manny his meal, and he told her to leave it on his nightstand. We all ate our food, and my wife and I put a movie in the DVD. The movie started up, and we started watching it. My wife and I agree that God did the following: we had both fallen asleep. After a time I heard my wife jump off the couch, which woke me up. She ran to Manny's room, and I heard nothing. I looked over at the television, and the movie had ended and the DVD menu was on the screen.

My wife suddenly came out of Manny's room and said, "Call 911."

I don't know why I said this, but out came, "Why? Is he dead?"

"Yes," she said.

I jumped off the couch and ran to Manny's room. He was on the floor faceup, and he wasn't breathing. I'll never forget the look on his face. I completely lost it. I couldn't dial 911. I had my cell phone in my hand, and the numbers just didn't make any sense. My poor wife had to run to the kitchen to make the call. The person tried to explain to my wife how to perform CPR on Manny. She told her, "No, Manny is gone. They let him die," referring to the doctors of course. Then my wife was told that help was on the way. In all this confusion, we didn't realize that my younger son had entered the Manny's room. He had seen his brother lying on the floor dead. He too had seen death in his brother's eyes.

Later my wife told me that when she entered the room, Manny was lying on his stomach like he was asleep. She thought he had a seizure and tapped him on his back. He didn't move. She then flipped him over. He had no color in his eyes; they had white haze, and his skin color was gray. She immediately realized that he was gone. She took Manny in her loving arms and took him off the bed. She held him in her arms as she sat on the floor. She had many emotions at once. She was angry at God. She said, "It should have been me instead. You took him too soon. I don't want to be here without him." She was so angry at God for taking him, when suddenly her vision was taken, and she heard a voice say that the best part of Manny was gone and she was holding his shell. Then her anger was taken away, and she felt peace. She placed Manny on the floor on his back and told him, "Don't worry, I'm going to be your voice from the grave. They are not going to get away with this." Then she yelled, "Call 911!"

I only hope and pray that Manny wasn't feeling worse than he made it sound. After all, he knew that the doctors didn't want to take care of him. I hope that he didn't figure that they won't do anything anyway and didn't seek medical care. Can you imagine what was going through his mind? Toward the end, Manny seemed to be swelling up. My wife told his doctors this fact, but it was pointless; they did nothing. He had also asked me, "Dad, is it normal to have a slight tremor in my hands?"

I told him maybe it was, because he was taking Dilantin. My wife also told his doctors this, but again it fell on deaf ears. I truly hope he didn't suffer. God only knows if he did or didn't.

Minutes later, the doorbell rang. It was our neighbor, who is a volunteer fireman. He was monitoring his scanner when he heard the call go out for Manny. When he heard the address, he immediately rushed over to our house. We let him in, and he went to Manny's room. He too immediately recognized that Manny was long gone. It was too late to do anything. He tried his best to calm us down. We told him how they neglected Manny and they let him die. He was very consoling, and he told us not to linger near Manny. "Let's sit down at the table and try to stay calm and wait for the police and ambulance."

A short time later, both the police and ambulance arrived. The EMS personnel went to Manny, and they saw he had passed, so they promptly left. The police treated the area as a crime scene, which I know is standard procedure, but at that time, it added insult to injury. They asked us questions, and we told them the story about what had happened to Manny. He was neglected by our health-care system, and his doctors let him die. They recognized that it wasn't a crime, but we couldn't go into Manny's room. I desperately wanted to take Manny in my arms and say my good-byes, but I wasn't allowed to. They called for the medical examiner, and we had to sit away from Manny's room. This was very disheartening.

The medical examiner arrived a short time later. He checked the scene, asked us the appropriate questions, and declared it to be a natural cause of death and that no foul play was involved. He then came to my wife and me and recommended to have an autopsy done. He told us that the system failed and that if we were going to sue, an autopsy should be done. We immediately agreed to the autopsy, and before he left, he said, "You get those bastards." Then they wrapped Manny in a body bag, and they removed his body from our home. This is something they made sure we didn't see.

I called my sister and told her that Manny had died she was distraught. I told her I couldn't find the courage to tell my parents. She told me she would do it. We agreed to let them sleep peacefully that evening and that she would tell them in the morning. My wife called her sister and told her the depressing news. Her sister spread the news to her family. So started the chain of phone calls that reached every member of both our families, hers and mine.

Levia and I started going through the grieving process. This process is, as you can imagine, not fun. The first stage we went through was denial. We couldn't believe that this tragedy had happened.

We also wanted to be alone and crawl under a rock. Then we went through a lot of anger, saying things like "Those damned doctors and those damned hospitals and the damned system," that type of stuff. Then came the should've, would've, could've. "We should have done this . . ." "If we would have done that . . ." "I could have done this . . ." This is what I call the "beat yourself up" stage. It's easy to say these things in hindsight, but the reality is, Manny was sent to a hospital that specializes in the type of condition he had. He was supposed to be in the best hands possible. They chose not to care for him adequately, waiting for the finances to come through. This is inexcusable; this should have never happened. But it did, and my family paid the ultimate price; we lost Manny, and he was precious to us.

Well, now the grueling task of arranging Manny's funeral was upon us. I have to say this is the hardest thing I ever had to do in my life. This is something that I don't wish on any parent, having to bury their child. It just goes against the grain; it isn't the way things are supposed to be. Children bury their parents, not the other way around. But thanks to a dysfunctional health-care system and greedy doctors, we now faced this process. We decided to go to our local funeral home.

So we went to Roma Funeral Home, and we met the directors, who were very compassionate. We told them Manny's horror story, and they were outraged. They treated us with courtesy, compassion, and respect. They made all the arrangement to make this process as painless as possible. Yes, we were distraught, but they handled every aspect of the funeral. We just told them what our wishes were, and they took care of everything. Then came the time where we had to pick out the casket. We were taken to the casket room. We entered a room that were full of caskets everywhere, all sizes and colors; it was surreal. Words cannot express what an emotional experience this is. I think this becomes the first time the reality of the situation sets in. My wife lost all composure at this point. She had to leave the room; she was crying and didn't want to see the caskets. It took a while for her to be able to return to the room and pick out Manny's casket. She was very angry.

Manny's favorite colors were red and black, so we chose a beautiful black casket. They said that they would recover the body from the medical examiner's office, which they did. The autopsy was done immediately, so we didn't have to wait for his remains. Now we had to pick a cemetery where we were going to lay Manny to rest. We chose a cemetery that was local. This way we could go visit his grave whenever we wanted to. The flower arrangements were made. We told the director that since Manny was a Star Wars enthusiast, we wanted to incorporate that theme in his flowers. She asked us to bring some Star Wars figures that could be set in his arrangements, which we supplied. Then she told us to bring a picture of Manny so that they could see how he looked in life so they could make him look that way now that he was gone. We were also asked to bring his clothes in which he was to be buried in.

Manny was not only a Stars Wars fan but he was also a Michael Jordan fan. He was also a WWF fan, and he had a jacket that he wore with the WWF logo and their top wrestlers that were printed on it. He constantly wore Michael Jordan's jersey with the number 23 on it and Jordan on the back. We asked the director if he could be buried in his jersey or if we had to get his "Sunday" clothes. She told us, "Listen, you can bury him in however you wanted." We wanted to bury Manny as he was. He wasn't a suit person. He was a black pants and jersey type, and that's the way we wanted him buried. So that was the way we buried him, in black pants and red jersey, and thus his favorite colors.

The day of the funeral came; he was to lie in state two days. We got dressed, and the family came to the house. We all went together to the funeral home. We arrived to where he laid in state, and the emotions of sorrow, anger, and denial set in; we all cried. There he was, lying in his casket, and he looked like he was sleeping. The first day our family and close friends and coworkers were present at the funeral. We all paid him our respects and spoke of him, and we remembered him as he was, saying to each other, "Remember this and remember that?" all with Manny's music playing in the background, music from Star Wars, his favorite songs from Metallica, etc. The time to go home came, and we said our good-byes. My wife said out loud, "Manny, get up, let's go home," and we went home, of course without him.

The next day was day 2 of the wake. We again went to the funeral home. We played his music and remembered him as he was. As time went by, more and more young people arrived, and the room was packed with people. I didn't know anyone. I went to my wife and asked her, "Honey, who are all these people?"

She answered, "These are Manny's friends and coworkers."

I was awestruck. I had no idea Manny had so many friends. Now Manny was given two rooms for his funeral, and it was standing room only. Not only that, there was a line of people, all Manny's friends, waiting to get in to pay their respects. You would swear that a celebrity had died.

The funeral director was amazed at the number of friends that had come to pay their respects. Person after person would come and tell us how Manny had touched their lives, how he would cheer them up when they were down, and how they all remembered his kindness and, most of all, his awesome smile. My wife and I were truly touched by the stories. They all reminded us something we already knew: he was a special person and how he put others first. He never ever judged a book by its cover. He saw the good in everything and everyone.

While all this was going on, there was this individual that was present, a person that wasn't particularly dressed well, not for a funeral anyway. He kind of gave me the impression that he was a hobo that worked his way into the wake. He kind of stood out; he looked like he didn't belong. I noticed him, and so did my wife. I was doing what Manny did not do. I was judging a book by its cover. This person, whose name I found out was Brother Steve, was trying to find Manny's parents. Finally he worked his way over to us.

I have to say, I thought he would smell bad, but he did not. When I looked into his eyes, I immediately felt a sense of peace, not only me, but my wife did also. I knew God had sent us an angel. He told us how he had a near-death experience. He told us that he had died for a brief time and that he saw the face of God. Then God shook his head and said no, then he was sent back to preach the truth. He told us that he had given up his belongings and served God, preaching his Word. He told us that Manny was in heaven and that he was at peace. He told us how Manny would pray with him every day before he started work. He would pray for us and all his friends. I had no idea that Manny did this.

My wife and I would often wonder why Manny would leave the house early to start work; now we knew why. He spoke praise of Manny, and I was so proud of my son. He was truly an angel on earth. After he said this, he walked away and continued through the crowd. After a short while, I was looking for him, and as God is my witness, he had disappeared, nowhere to be found. Now I'm not saying he vanished into thin air, because I didn't witness that. What I am saying is, one minute he was among the crowd. Then a short time later, when I was looking for him, he was just no longer present. I never saw him again.

A short time later, my younger son lost his composure. He had enough with the funeral, and he wanted to go home. The next day was Manny's burial, so I thought it was probably best to take him home. I told my wife what was happening and told her I was taking him home. I told her I wasn't going to leave him by himself and that I was going to stay with him. She agreed with me. I said my good-byes, and I left the wake. My son calmed down, and shortly after arriving home, like a small child, he fell asleep. My wife came home a short time later. A neighbor that was at the wake had driven her home.

Then we found out that the Wendy's that my son worked at had closed for the day and lowered the flag to half-mast. They waved the flag this way for a week in tribute to Manny. I would like to thank them for this honor. They did all they could to help him; they even got him health insurance. Unfortunately, the preexisting condition was in effect, and the insurance he finally did get at the end did him no good. Not because of Wendy's, but because of the insurance industry. This was before Obamacare changed and made the preexisting condition illegal. If it wasn't for this provision, he might have been taken care of. I pray to God that this provision never comes into effect again.

The next day had arrived; we were going to bury Manny. This was the last day we were going to see Manny's face in physical form. The weather was weird. It rained, it snowed, and the sky was overcast. The limousine came to get us and took us to the funeral home. There we were again, and there he was lying in his coffin. The reality of never seeing him again started setting in. We played some songs that we dedicated to him. The first song we played was a song by Josh Groban called "To Where You Are." Then we played a song by Beth Hart called "I'll Stay with You." Levia dedicated this song to Manny when he had first gotten sick. Then we played a song that was one of his favorites, and it represented him and the way he lived. This song was from Metallica called "Nothing Else Matters." We played them, and tears ran down our faces. We said our good-byes to Manny.

We took the CD that was played during the wake and put it in the coffin. Levia put a shaver in his pocket because he always wanted to be clean cut; he hated excessive hair. Then we took his WWF jacket that he always wore. We placed it over him like you would a blanket. We also put his gizmo stuffy in his coffin; this he had since his childhood, and he loved it.

The funeral director asked for some pallbearers to carry the coffin to the hearse. I of course stayed. Levia said, "I'll help carry him. I carried him for nine months and gave him life, and I'll carry him now in death to his resting place." My brother-in-law was another, and his close cousin, my nephew. The casket was closed, a really tough thing to watch. We picked up the casket, and we walked him over to the hearse and placed him in ever so gently.

Several floral arrangements were taken and placed in the flower car. We got into the limousine, and everyone else into their cars. Everyone turned their headlights and four-way flashers on, and so started the procession. We drove around the neighborhood where we live and passed our house, as is customary. Several neighbors were outside and bowed their heads in respect, and off we went to the cemetery.

We arrived, and the grave had already been dug up. The sky was still overcast, but no rain or snow was falling. There was a lowering device over the grave to lower the casket. We again carried his casket and placed it onto the device. Everyone got out and gathered around the grave. My wife's sister had twenty-five white balloons that were to be let loose when the casket was to be lowered. We asked everyone to watch the balloons and not the casket until they were no longer visible. The deacon said some prayers, some eulogies were said, and as the casket started lowering, the balloons were released. Everyone present watched the balloons as they rose into the sky.

Then several things happened. One of the balloons kind of lingered and flew lower than the others. Then the clouds broke and the sun came out and the rays of sunshine shone behind the balloons. Then several doves flew across the sky. We watched the balloons until the clouds took them and they could no longer be seen. My wife and I believe that the balloon that lingered was Manny's spirit that didn't want to leave us. The clouds that opened and let the sun shine was heaven opening up, and the doves flying across the sky was God's way of telling us that Manny was now in heaven. By the time the balloons disappeared, the casket was now at the bottom of the grave. We took roses, and we threw them on top of Manny's casket one by one; everyone present did the same. We lingered a bit, but we left but a piece of our hearts right there in Manny's grave. Our angel was gone; only his memories remain.

My wife wrote letter in her journal to Manny, and this is what she wrote:

> Manuel Nickie Lanza Jr. Born July 9, 1980. January 6, 2005 was the day I died, my first born died, because doctors told themselves that his life wasn't worth saving. My child was the best; he finished school and worked hard as a chef. He never did drugs or drank. He helped my husband and me in more ways than one. How can a mother just go on living when her child has been taken away or left to die? I keep hearing take one day at a time. That's easier said than done. I miss him so much. Manny had the heart of Gold and he worried about everyone but himself. I pray to God and hope he died without pain. Nobody understood me like my son. He was always there for me. He would ask me; what's wrong mom? I can see it in your face; I didn't want him to know that I was fighting with the hospital and social service on the phone for his life. My God we grew up together he was my best friend. I am having trouble sleeping. Since that day when I

close my eyes at night all I see is death in my son's face, no mother should see this. Dear God we were so much alike, both hardheaded, with a love for life. Please can someone wake me up from this nightmare and give me back my son. My life will never be the same! The days are going by and I still live at that time and day with a heavy heart full of pain. Can somebody tell me how to live without Manny, who was the heart of this family. I can't tell if I'm coming or going. Now the little peace I have is when I'm asleep, but as soon as I awaken my nightmare begins again. Knowing that he is gone and that he is never coming back. I will never hear him laugh or go for walks which he loved to do; or when I just needed a hug he would always be there for me. I will never rest on this earth until they pay for letting him die. Why do doctors play God? All I can say to you my son is, sorry! That this happened to you. You will never be forgotten, I love you always. Mom.

I also wrote him a little note. It's one of the things that you do to deal with the grief. I was and am still missing him; I suppose I always will until we are united again. Here is what I wrote:

My dear son Manny, I love you more than words can say. My heart yearns for your precious smile. But now you're free, my son. You are no longer burdened by life's woes. You can now do all that you wanted to. I promise you that you will live in my heart forever; because you were (are) a great son. You never caused me any grief and I thank you for all the help that you gave me. You are the "best"; you are the "man". You are now my son, an angel. So spread your wings and soar, live free and enjoy; for I know that you are in better place than me. Until we meet again don't ever forget I always have and always will love you. Love always your loving father Rey.

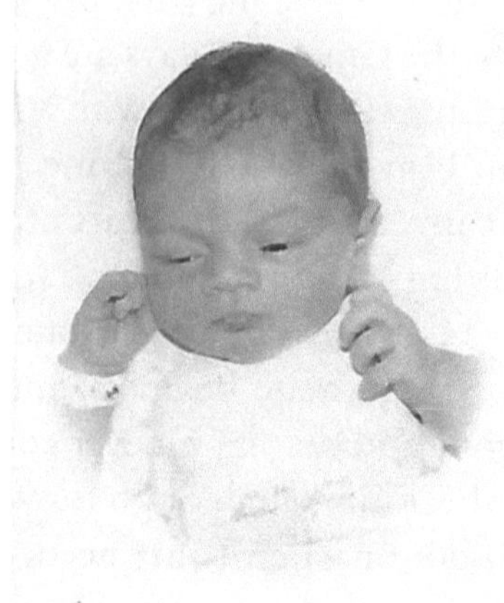

Manny newborn

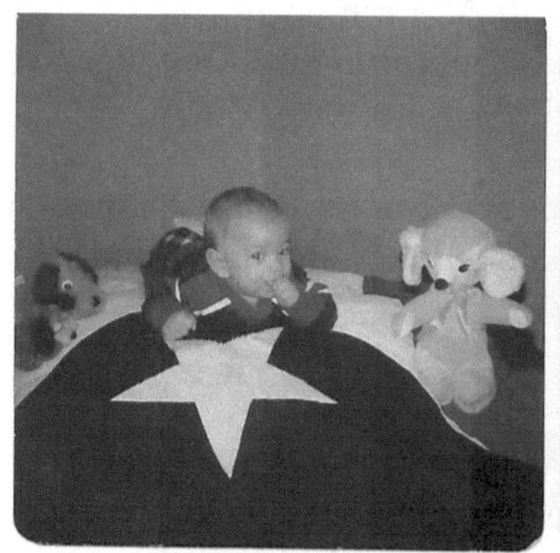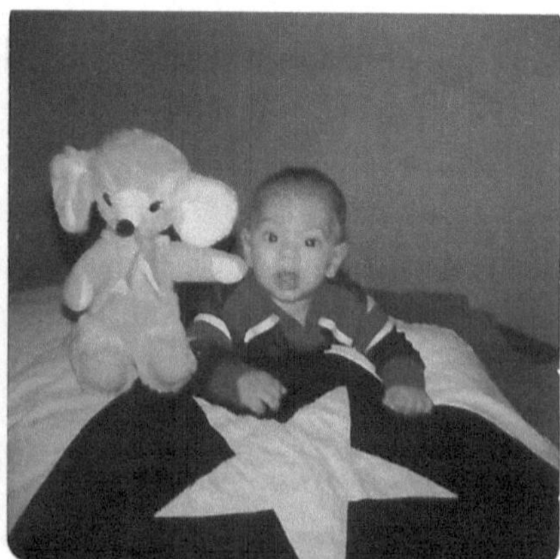

Manny when he became part of my life

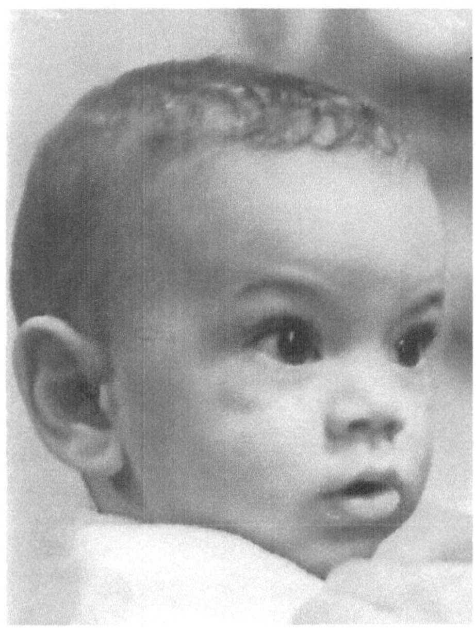

Manny at a year old

Before I get into the rest of the story, I want to tell you a little about Manny. He was born Manuel Nickie Lanza Junior on July 9, 1980, in Elmhurst Hospital in Queens, New York. He weighed seven pounds ten ounces and measured twenty-two and one-fourth inches. His biological mother is Levia Garcia, who later became my wife. His biological father was Manuel Lanza. Their relationship ended after Levia was six months pregnant. He was never to become a part of Manny's life.

I met Manny's mother, Levia, on May 26, 1981. I was sitting at the local pizzeria, when Levia entered. I was a very shy individual, and so she took the first step. She walked over, took off my glasses, and said, "You have beautiful eyes." For me it was love at first sight. We have been together ever since. That was when not only Levia but also Manny became part of my life, something that I never regretted. Then on July 9, 1981, which was Manny's first birthday, as circumstances and fate would dictate, Levia and I started living together. We were two seventeen-year-old kids ourselves, raising a baby. We started living with my parents. At that time my sister was getting married and was leaving the nest to start her new life with her husband. Manny was to fill the void of my sister leaving. He made the transition easier for my parents, and they loved him always.

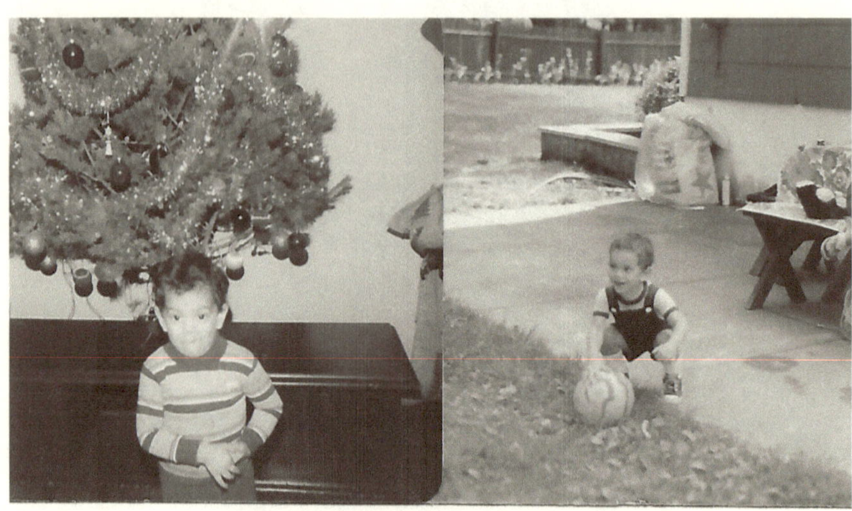

Manny at Christmas and on his second Birthday

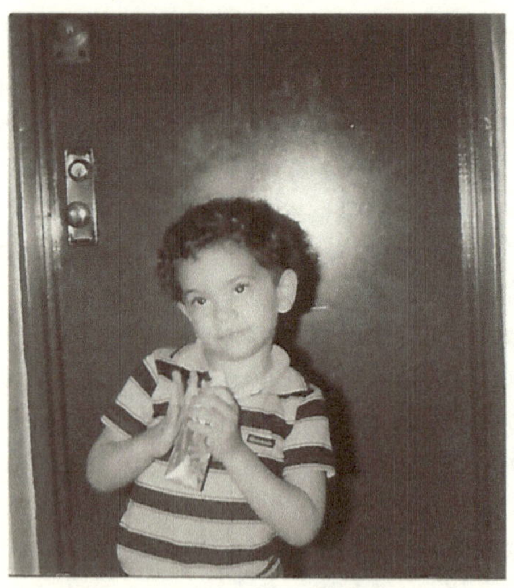

Our little Angel notice the halo

Manny was more like a younger brother than a son. As time went by and he grew, he became more and more like a friend. Everywhere we went he was with us. My wife and I always said it was Rey, Levia, and Manny. Like three peas in a pod, we went through life with all its ups and downs together. Despite external forces such as jealous friends and acquaintances trying to break us up, we survived the test of time. You would figure a couple so young would never make it, but we defied all the odds and were a happy family.

Manny was a happy baby. The sounds of him laughing, which he did often, brought joy into our lives. I honestly never thought that was possible, but even from an early age, he always brought a smile to my face. We enjoyed his curiosity experiencing things for the first time. I enjoyed watching him; play his imagination was endless. I remember one Christmas he was given a stuffed bunny, which he loved from the moment he received it. This bunny was to become his pillow, and it was the only pillow he would use. He used it until the material became paper thin and it was no longer repairable. When the time to get rid of it came, we had to have a funeral for his bunny. This was what Manny wanted, so we buried the bunny in our yard.

We had three dogs early in Manny's life. The eldest dog was a little dog named Jill. The second eldest was Lobo; he was a mixed-breed dog. The youngest of the three was a Husky-type dog, and her name was Candy. This was Manny's favorite dog, and she was very gentle with him. She seemed to have sort of a motherly instinct with him. When he would wake up earlier than the rest of us, we would always find him under the kitchen table, resting his head on her. Candy never seemed to mind this; it was almost like she thought of him like her puppy. She was very protective of Manny, and he loved her so much. No matter what Manny did to her, such as hugging or playing with her, she was always very gentle with him. She was like a K-9 babysitter to him.

Manny was a healthy baby; he never had any illnesses aside from the usual common cold or belly aches and the usual maladies that affect us all. He went through the stages of a baby, learning to walk and to talk. Manny walked on the tips of his toes, a habit he would carry until his death. His heels never touched the ground. He was a happy baby, and he was always smiling and laughing. He brought joy to our household. Levia, who is a Pat Benatar fan and accomplished singer, would always sing her songs to him, so every time he heard the songs on the radio, he would always say his mother's name, Levia. Since he was young he would say Eeya. Time went by, and the day came for Manny to start school.

Manny started elementary school, and he was looking forward to it. He wanted to make new friends, and he wanted to learn to read and write. We of course as parents were a bit nervous. This marked the first time he wouldn't be at our side. Our fears were unjustified; he didn't cry the way most children do. He did the opposite. He went in and immediately started making friends; he just had a way of doing this. He was happy, and he looked forward every day in going to school, and he started learning how to write the alphabet, which he practiced every day.

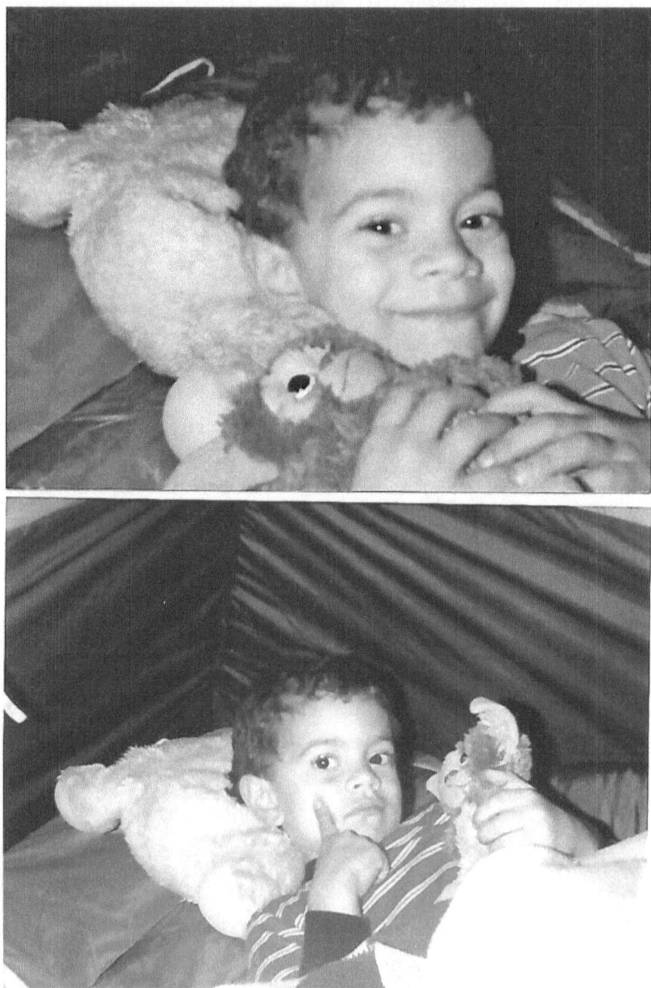

His two favorite things a rabbit stuffy that
was to become his pillow and Gizmo

Manny enjoyed school. He loved being with other children his age. He never wanted to miss school even when he wasn't feeling well. In fact, Manny received many awards for perfect attendance and many other awards every year. He took pride in doing so. He was soft-spoken and well mannered, a trait he would carry all his life. He was liked not only by his teachers but by his peers as well. Manny had a way of getting under your skin, not in an irritating way, but in a way that made you love him. This was also a trait he would carry all his life.

Manny wasn't judgmental. He accepted a person for who they were. He got promoted every year, and he always did what was expected of him not only in school but also in life in general.

Then the time came that we moved from our house in Levittown and went to Babylon. Manny was a bit upset that he wasn't going to see his friends. We told him that he was going to make new friends. He knew he would; he was just was going to miss his current ones. That summer he spent his time with us, settling into a new home, and as always, he made the best of the situation at hand. We made his room extra special, and he added his touches the way any child does. He also enjoyed the large yard that we now had at the new place. We entertained him that summer, taking him to the beach, which he loved. He especially loved playing in the sand with his toys. We also took him to the amusement park, to the petting zoo, and to the movies and camping, which he especially loved. Manny loved taking family trips, and he loved going to Roscoe, New York, where we usually went camping. He really loved the mountains and the river, which was right next to the campsite. He was enjoying himself, but he was missing his friends.

Many of our summer vacations were spent in Florida. Manny loved it there; after all, Disney World was there. I remember the first time we took him there. He was in complete awe. He just loved all the Disney characters and was absolutely fascinated by them. He loved going on the all the rides and didn't seem to mind waiting on the lines that are usual in Disney World.

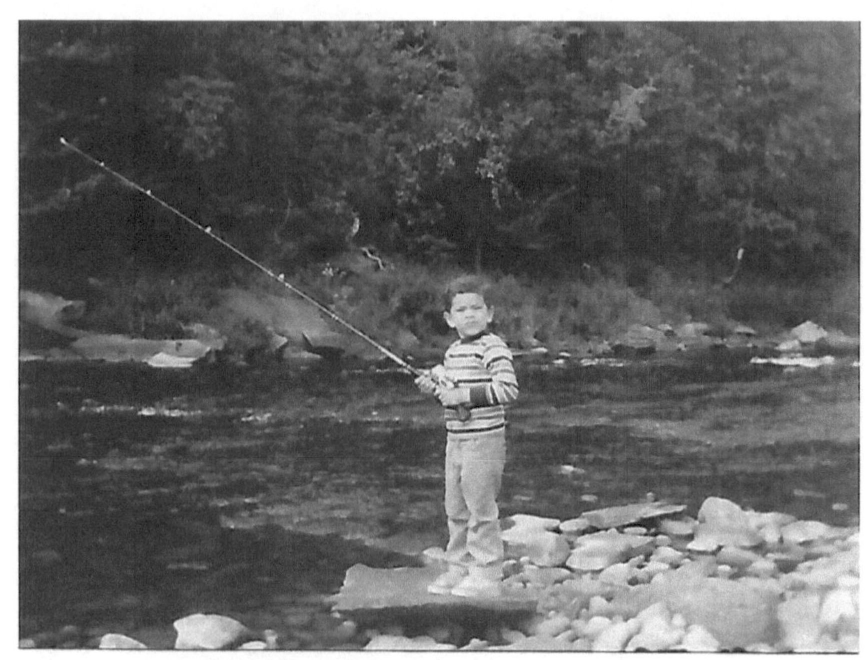

Fishing at the Beaverkill River in Roscoe

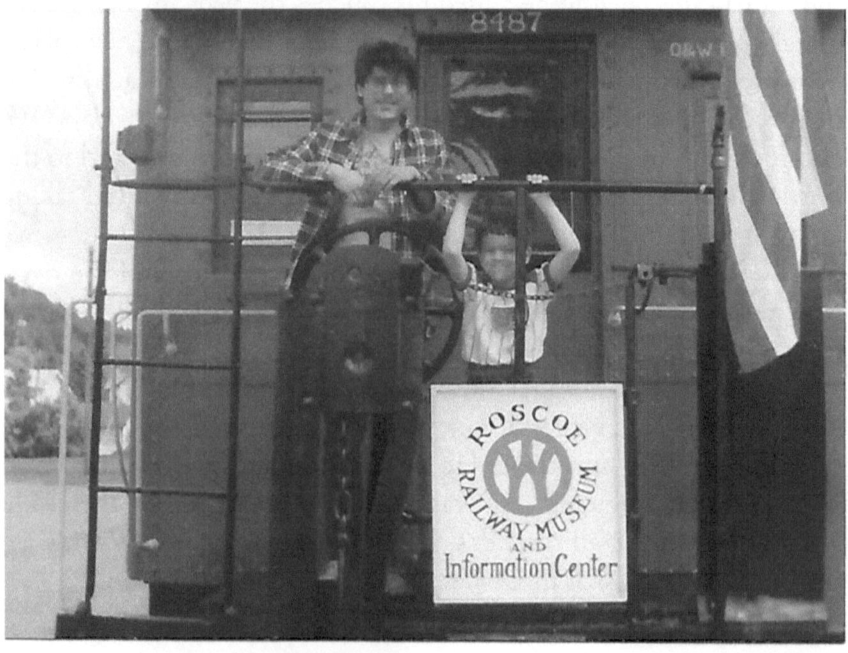



Manny and me in Roscoe

The summer ended, and again it was time to start school. He was going to start the second grade. Most children would be nervous going to a new school, but not Manny. He couldn't wait to start; he wanted to make new friends. The bus came to pick him up, and he left with great enthusiasm. He of course made several friends on his first day. Like I've said, he just had this outgoing personality, and he just was able to make friends easily. I wish I had this gift. He definitely got this trait from his mother; she's the same way. When he got home, he couldn't wait to tell us about his new friends. We of course were very proud of him. He went to school every day and ended the year, again getting awarded for perfect attendance. We stayed in Babylon for about three years, and he went to the Babylon district until the fourth grade.

The video game era had arrived, and being young, I was fascinated by them. The Atari game system came out, and I of course got one. Manny was also fascinated by the video games, and soon we would play together. At first his skills weren't so good, but as time went by, he would become better and better at it. His skills got so good that eventually he would surpass my skills and he became very hard to beat. Manny played video games all through his life, and he had become so skilled at it that he would always win. Manny had the heart of a winner, and he would always excel in whatever he set his heart and mind to. He played all the genres of video games: Atari, Nintendo, Super Nintendo, and so on. He played them, and he was happy doing so.

Then Levia got pregnant, and we decided that it was time we had our own place. We were renting our place up to this point. We bought an old house in Bay Shore that was on a dead-end street. It had plenty of yard space, and I thought this was a good place to expand our family. The house needed work, but I was willing to fix it to make it work for us.

Manny was excited to move to our own home. He was going to miss his friends of course, and he had to start in a new school again. He was going on ten years of age, and he was promoted to the fifth grade. We rented a truck, and with several of our friends, we moved into our own home.

When Manny turned ten years old, my second son was born. Manny was happy to have a younger brother. He was proud to be the older brother. He loved him and was always watching over him. You would figure that after ten years of being the only child he would be jealous, but he wasn't. This wasn't Manny's way; he accepted his brother from the beginning. The age difference was a deficit at first. After all, ten years was a lot, especially through his teenage years. But as time went on, he became close to his brother, and his brother was getting close to him. They were bonding. This was all taken away when Manny died; this devastated his younger brother.

Then the time again came for him to start school. As usual he was excited in making new friends. As was the normal for him, he made friends on the first day. I am still amazed at how easy he made friends. He finished elementary school and started junior high soon after. He zipped his way through that, getting his usual awards along the way. He never wanted to miss school and always wanted to improve himself in the learning process. He never wanted to fail, and he never did. Then he started high school, and he went to Bay Shore High School.

Manny went through high school again, being very responsible and never wanting to miss classes. Again he received awards for perfect attendance. He also received the awards for the Breakfast of Champions several months in a row for several years. This was a reward where the high school would recognize the achievements of students and they would get a breakfast in their honor at the local diner. He was also honored in the Renaissance Program, which honored academic excellence. We of course were proud of him. Manny never caused us any grief. He never smoked, he never drank alcohol, and he never did drugs. In fact, he would participate in the DARE program at school. This was a program that the local police department would do to promote students to be drug- and alcohol-free, and he took pride to be part of it. He would participate in events like when the April 19, 1995, terrorist attack in Oklahoma City took place. Manny was involved in a fund-raiser for the victims of that attack. These were things he was very proud of.

Then came the day when Bay Shore High School was figuring out careers for their students. Manny decided that he would become a chef, and he was enrolled in the BOCES course that he was to start the following year. This was a two-year course that was to be followed by an internship program. He would start this program in his junior year. He caught a lot of slack that summer from some of the neighborhood kids that he was going to cooking school. You know how cruel teenagers can be; they tried to embarrass Manny.

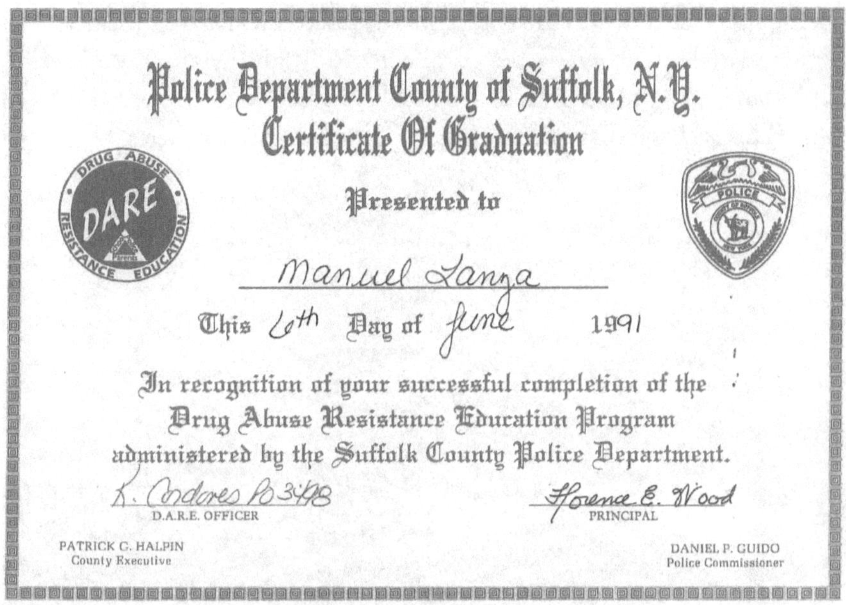


This is Dare Certificate Of Graduation

One day Manny came into the house a little dejected by the insults. I asked him what was wrong. He told me that the kids were saying that he was taking a girls' course. He told me some were taking auto mechanics or auto body or welding courses, telling him these were manly courses. I told him that becoming a chef was a noble profession. "The best cooks in the world are men," I said. I told him that everyone has to eat every day and that chefs are well respected. "Those kids will be coming to your restaurant when they are hungry, you'll see," I said. "Then you will be respected and admired by them, I promise you."

He got the message, and he never again felt ashamed for becoming a chef. In fact, he was quite proud, and when the kids said the insults, it didn't bother him and they stopped. He used everything I had told him as his defense, and he was never bothered again.

Manny's graduation day came, and he was getting ready for the day. We were proud of him. What parent wouldn't be? We all dressed up in our Sunday best. It was a beautiful day, and his ceremony was to be held outdoors. He dressed in his red cap and gown, and he left slightly before us. We went to the high school field, and we sat in our chairs. My parents were with us, and we waited for the ceremony to start. The graduation theme then started, and the graduates marched out and slowly filled their appropriate seats. It was a beautiful ceremony, and Manny received his diploma. He was officially a high school graduate. We were very proud of him. This was the first of three graduations he graced us with.

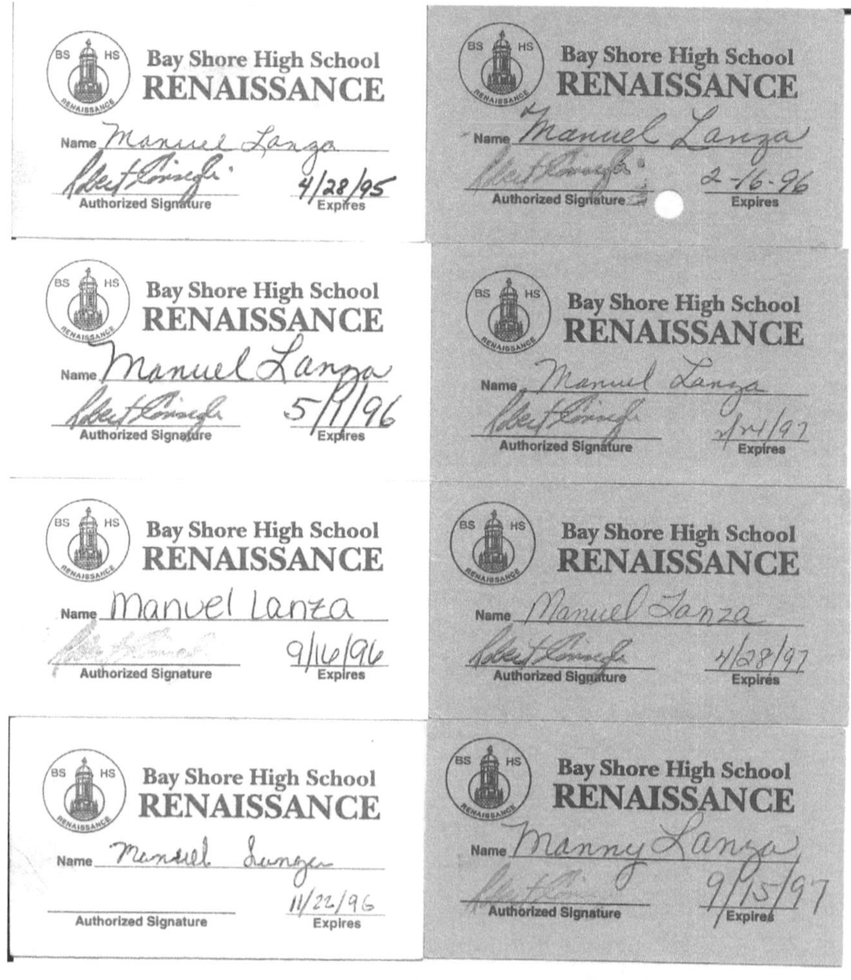


These were some of his Renaissance cards. These gave him certain privileges and discounts at our local stores

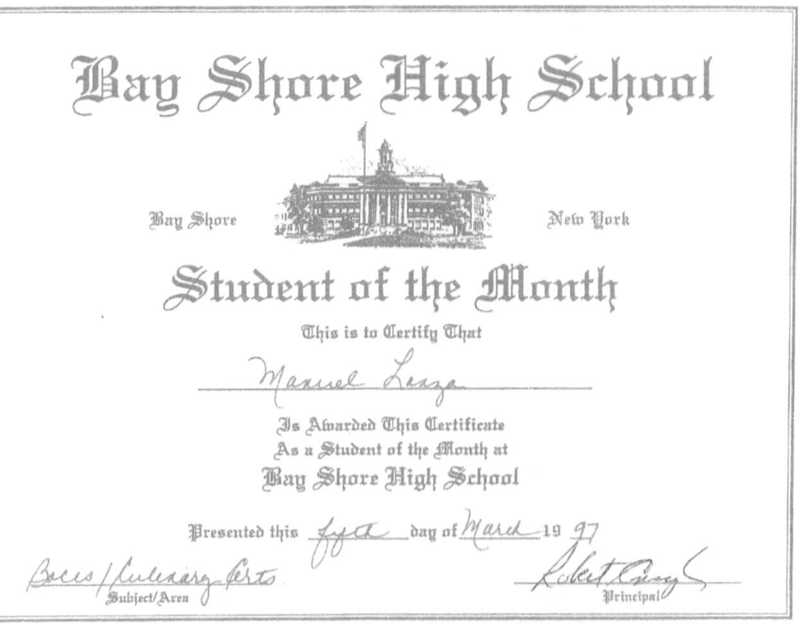


This is an award he received for Student
of the Month in March of 1997

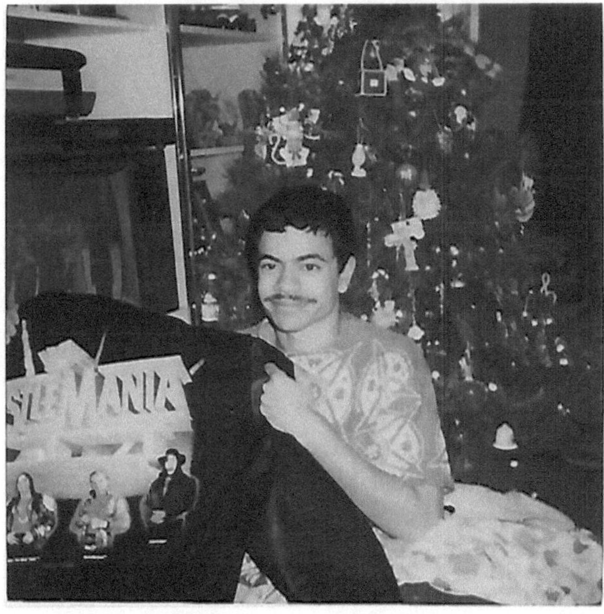

This is his WWF jacket that he wore all the time

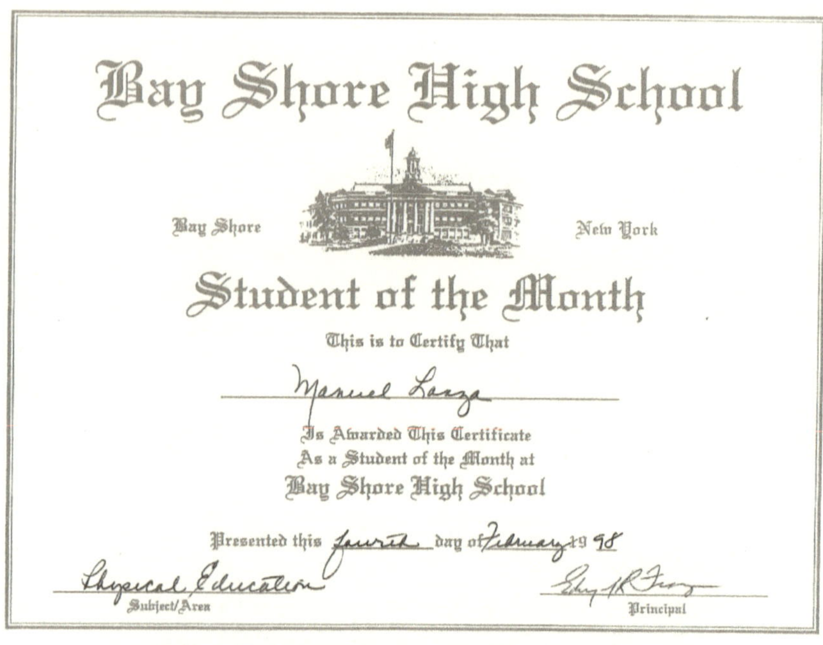

This is another award for Student of the Month February 1998

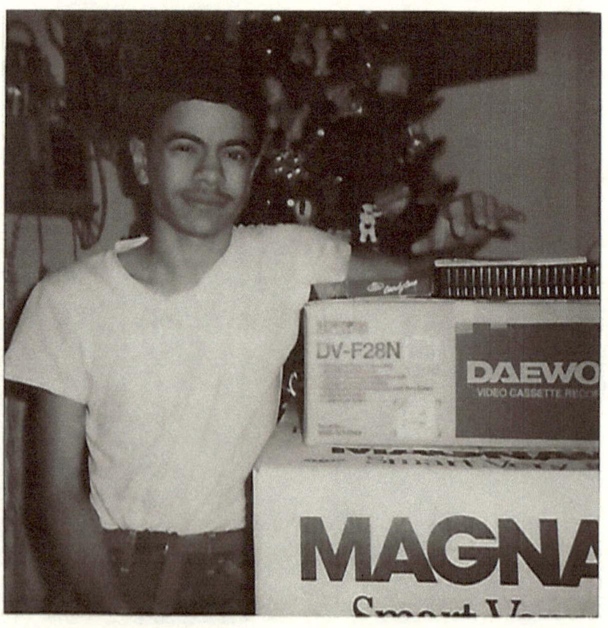

Manny with a new TV and VCR at Christmas

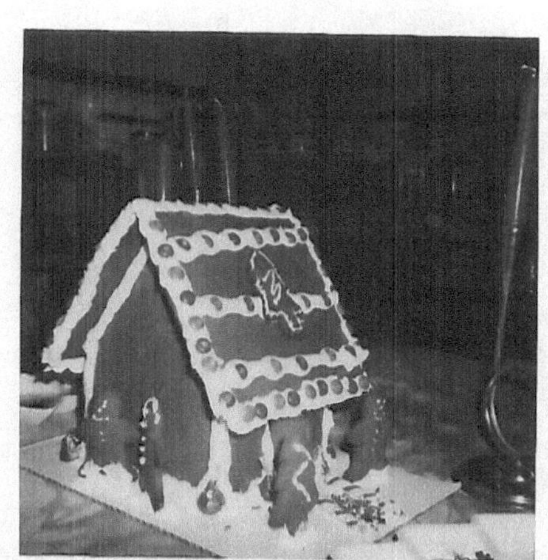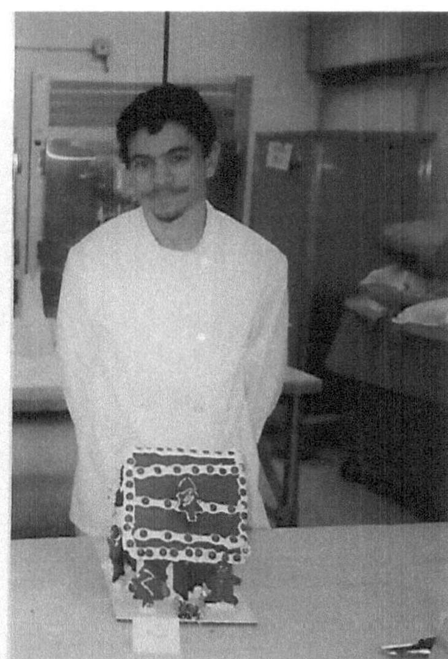

Manny at BOCES with his Gingerbread House

Now it was time to graduate from BOCES, and this was the second graduation that we had the pleasure of attending. It was a smaller ceremony, but it was an honor just the same. Manny again got ready and was excited that he had graduated and was going to get his two-year degree. We attended the ceremony, and it was beautiful. Manny got his diploma, and we were so proud of him. His two-year diploma was for culinary arts and restaurant management.

Manny graduated high school, and he also graduated from BOCES. He had two years of cooking under his belt. Then he decided to go to the Culinary Academy in Westbury, New York. He had an internship program, which was part of the curriculum, and he worked at the Olive Garden. They decided to keep him employed after the internship was over. He graduated from there and got his degree as a professional chef. He was proud of this, but not as proud as we were of him. He stayed at the Olive Garden for four years until we moved farther out east and his commute became overbearing. Normally, this wouldn't be the case, but now we realize that he must have been feeling weary because he had an AVM that we didn't know about yet.

Then he asked us if we minded terribly if he worked at Wendy's for now because the travel was getting to him. We told him, "Of course not. We are proud of you and whatever you do." So he started work at Wendy's and became the manager's right-hand man. Manny was awarded Employee of the Month and then became Employee of the Year, which was the year just before his death, 2004.

Manny was very responsible when it came to his work ethics. He always made himself available if needed. The only day that he wouldn't work was on Monday. Manny just hated Mondays. I agree with him there. He would tell his bosses that he would be available any day except Monday. None of his bosses minded this because he would always work weekends, which are the "busy" days. Many times he would get up earlier than usual to go to work early or stay late if needed. If he was called in because someone had called in sick, he would always say, "OK, Boss, I'll be in as soon as possible." Then he would get ready and go in to work. His bosses always knew that they could depend on Manny.

I remember once when he was working at the Olive Garden and he had come home earlier than usual. He came into the house, and he seemed to be irritated. Obviously something was bothering him. He was always so cheerful, and to see him irritated was not normal for him. We asked him, "Manny, what is wrong? Did something happen?"

"I'm so angry at one of the assistant managers right now," he said.

We were stunned Manny was angry at someone. This was very unusual. Then he told us his story.

"Today was very busy day, and I was about to prepare a chicken cutlet parmesan entrée. After I cooked the chicken and went to put it on the plate, I accidentally dropped it and it fell to the floor. The assistant manager of course was present in the kitchen. When he witnessed that I was going to throw the chicken out, he freaked out. He wanted me to continue to serve it to the customer. I told him, 'No way, I'm not serving that. It fell on the floor.' The manager didn't care. He insisted, he said it is very busy. I told him, 'This is not the way I was trained to run a kitchen. This is my kitchen, and I will run it properly.' We went back and forth, and since he kept insisting to serve this contaminated chicken, I took off my apron and threw the chicken in the garbage. I told him, 'It's my permit on the wall, not yours,' then I quit."

I told him, "You did the right thing. That is exactly what you are supposed to do. You can't serve that piece of meat to the customer."

"I know," he said, "but now I have no job."

I told him, "Don't worry. You did right. You stuck to your guns and made the proper decision, good for you. Don't worry, you'll find another job." I saw the sense of relief in his expression.

Then to his surprise, the very next day the general manager called our house. He wanted to talk to Manny. Manny took the phone and started talking to the manager. Evidently, she knew Manny and immediately realized that if Manny walked off the job, there had to be a very good reason. Manny told her what had happened, and she agreed with him. She told him that he done the right thing. Turns out that the assistant manager only told her that Manny just got up and quit; he didn't say anything about the contaminated chicken. She knew that had to be a reason, and now she knew. The assistant manager was fired, and Manny was asked to return to work. He was very happy to hear that he still had a job. He couldn't wait to tell us. Then I told him, "See? I told you that you handled the matter correctly."

He carried this ethic over to Wendy's. The following is a letter from Manny's boss, Joe, from Wendy's. This shows how dedicated and responsible he was. It also tells of how they wanted to move him up to management position. Manny loved and respected his bosses.

To Whom It May Concern,

In the 3 years I knew and worked with Manny I saw in him some pretty rare qualities. In the fast food business you don't often come across younger people with the combination of a very good work ethic, a drive to do their personal best and a pleasant, helpful demeanor. Manny had all these qualities and much more.

His overall performance earned him an Employee of the Month award, and his ongoing commitment to quality earned him our 2004 Employee of the Year award. His continuing effort to broaden his knowledge and sharpen his skills was an inspiration to many.

Whenever called upon Manny rose to the occasion, whether it was coming to work on his day off, staying later than scheduled, or leaving early during slower business periods Manny's response was always the same, "Whatever you need boss." He was a great contributor to the overall success of our operation.

We often talked about Manny taking the next step from crew to shift-supervisor, which I'm sure he would have met with much success. Unfortunately this never came to fruition.

It greatly saddens me to write this letter for which it is intended. The tragedy that has befallen the Lanza family has also deeply affected our Wendy's family here in Shirley.

Manny had and still has many friends here. Not just co-workers and bosses, we were truly friends. He also touched, if only in a small way, the lives of many guests he served here. He is and always will be missed.

I'm thankful to have known and worked with Manny as are many others here. I'm also thankful to have the opportunity know his family and be embraced by their love and kindness.

I hope you find the content of this letter to be helpful in appreciating and understanding the impact this young man's life had on me and many others here. I remain as always at your disposal should any further information be needed of Manny's time here at Wendy's.

Respectfully,
Joseph R. Carthe
Assistant Mgr. Wendy's Shirley

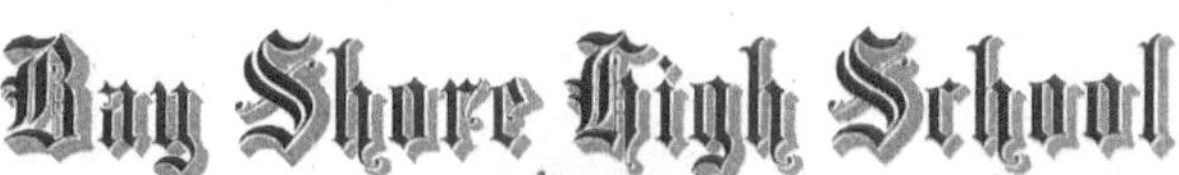
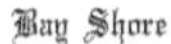
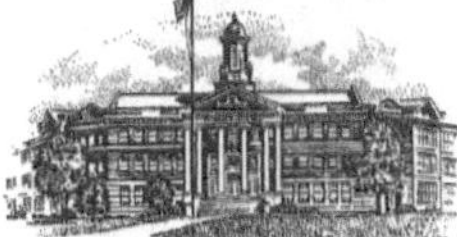
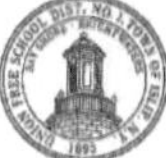

# Bay Shore High School

Bay Shore                    New York

This is to certify that

## Manuel Lanza

has satisfactorily completed a course of study prescribed by the Board of Education for Bay Shore High School and approved by the Regents of the University of the State of New York, and in recognition thereof is awarded this

## Diploma

Given this twenty-sixth day of June nineteen hundred and ninety-eight.

President, Board of Education

Principal of High School                    Superintendent of Schools

This was his High School diploma

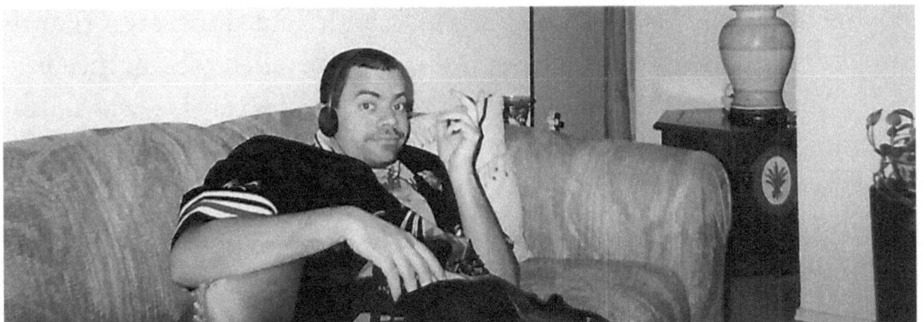

Manny's famous expression one his brother does today

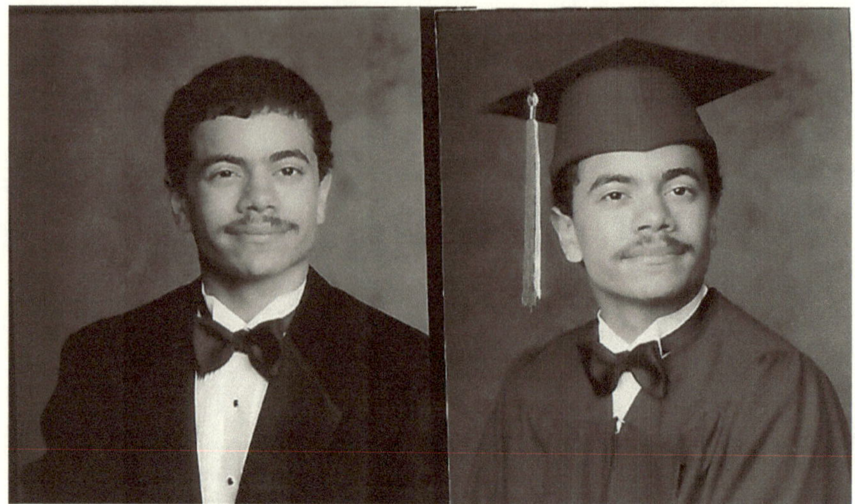

Manny in his tuxedo and cap and gown

Manny became quite interested in basketball, mostly because of his admiration of Michael Jordan and the Chicago Bulls, which was the greatest team at that time. I used to rib him about liking a Chicago team when he was a New Yorker. That didn't bother him, and he would tell me that the New York Knicks were losers. "They suck," he would say, and you know what? He was right; they did. Every televised Bulls game he would watch. He used to put his basketball, which carried the Bulls logo, and place it on top of his waste paper basket that also had the Bulls logo on it, and since it was slightly smaller in diameter than a basketball, it sat perched on top nicely.

Anyway, he became quite the basketball player. He was tall by this time; he was six feet one inch, taller than me. He was taller than his friends, and like everything else he did, he excelled in basketball. He would play and beat all his friends even when he spotted them points. He would play two against one, him being the one of course; three against two, again him being at the disadvantage, and he very rarely lost a game. So again he gained respect for being the best player among all his friends. Something I instilled in him, I always told him, "No matter what you do, be the best you can at it." This advice he lived by all the days of his short life.

Manny also liked hockey. His favorite team was the New York Islanders. He would watch the televised games when they were on. He loved watching those games. He would also wear the Islander jersey while he cheered them on. I was also an Islander fan, and many times we would watch them together, cheering when one of our team scored, jeering when the opposing team scored or we got a bad call from one of the officials. These are very fond memories that I will cherish forever.

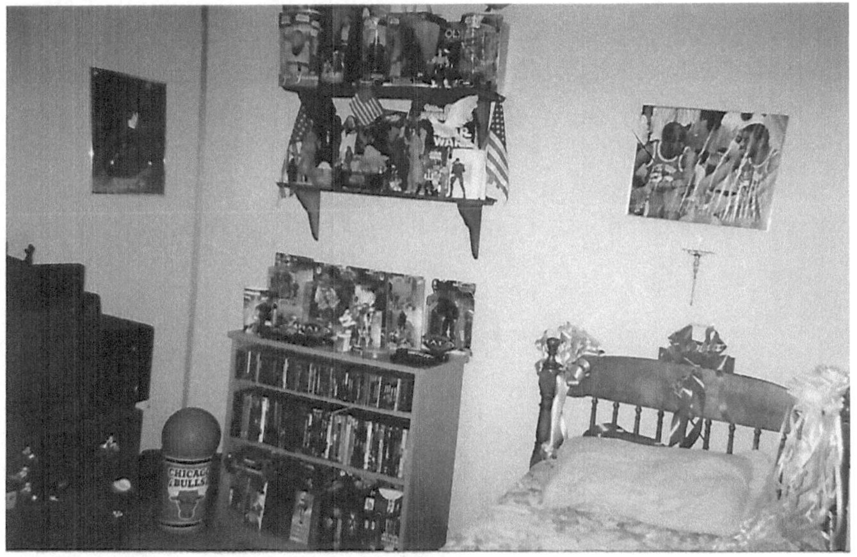

Manny's Room as left when he passed

He also loved professional wrestling. He loved to watch them every Monday when it was televised. He would often take his wrestling action figures and have them out during the matches. Manny actually thought the matches were real. I would tell him that the matches were not real and that the wrestlers were only acting. He would argue with me, saying, "No way, they are real." I never pushed the issue much because I remember when I was younger and I used to watch it, I too thought that it was real. It was later that I learned otherwise. So I let Manny live out his fantasy in believing that it was real. He enjoyed it, so why mess up his fun?

Manny also admired Bruce Lee, a person I also admired. He loved to watch his movies over and over, and I would watch them with him. Manny, for some reason, said that he would live like Bruce Lee.

He would say that he was never getting married, that he was never having kids, and that he was dying young. In hindsight, I wonder if he had a premonition, eerie, to say the least. His mother would always say to him, "You can't leave me. You don't want to leave your mama."

Manny also liked Marvel comic books; he loved all the different characters. He liked Spiderman, the Fantastic Four, the Punisher, Wolverine, and most of the others. He would get all the comic books and movies and keep track of the upcoming movies. He knew all the dates of the releases, and he would tell us when they were coming to the theaters. He had a way of finding out information about the upcoming movies. Manny was a kid at heart when he got a new movie or game. He would come to the kitchen table with the movie, and while he was eating, he would look at his new movie case. When I remember all these things about him, it brings a smile to my face. We miss him dearly

# Eastern Suffolk B.O.C.E.S.

## Career Education Division

BOARD OF COOPERATIVE EDUCATIONAL SERVICES

DISTRICT #1                    SUFFOLK COUNTY

*Be it known that*

## Manuel N. Lanza

*has satisfactorily completed training and*

*instruction in the curriculum area of*

## Culinary Arts / Restaurant Operations Management - Two Year

*Given at Suffolk County, New York, 1998*

_______________________
Executive Officer

_______________________
President
Board of Cooperative Educational Services

_______________________
Executive Director
Instructional Programs

This is his BOCES  diploma

# Culinary Academy of Long Island, Inc.

Be it known that

## Manuel N. Lanza

has successfully completed the course in

## Professional Cooking with Internship Program

and is awarded this

## Certificate

Granted at Westbury, New York

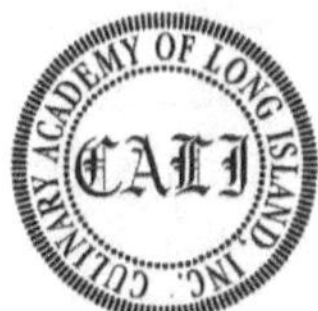

April 2, 1999
Date

Michael Lentt
Director

This is his Culinary Academy diploma

# Culinary Academy of Long Island

is proud to award this

## Certificate of Merit

to

### Manuel N. Lanza

for outstanding accomplishment and performance in

### Attendance

April 2, 1999
Date

*Michael Lentt*
Director

This is his Certificate of Merit for Attendance

Manny was a big Star Wars fan. He knew everything there was to know about the saga. He collected just about everything that came out. His uncle, Levia's younger brother Junior, would start him on his collection and his love for the series. Junior gave him his collection of original action figures as well as the original large figures of the characters. He also gave him the original ships like the *Millennium Falcon* and the X-wing fighter. Manny also collected comic books, Marvel of course; he didn't care much about DC comics. He collected movies and video game characters, figures, mostly from Nintendo. He collected Chicago Bulls and Islander memorabilia. He of course cherished them, and we still have his collection today.

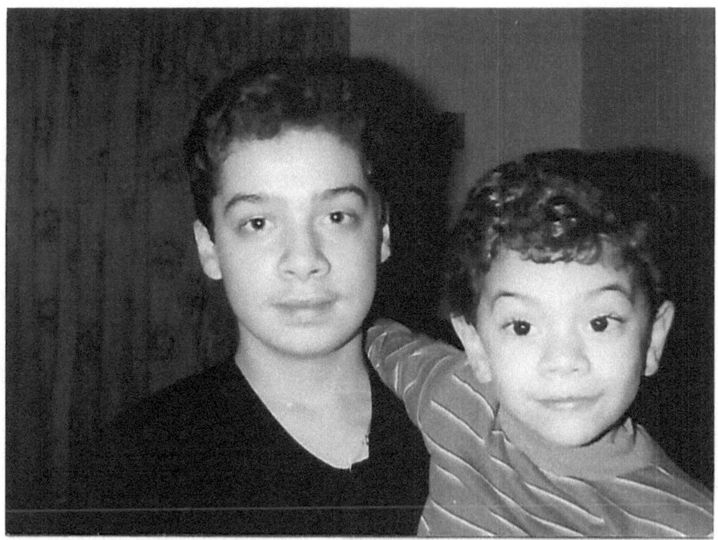

Manny with his uncle Junior

He owned and watched all the movies, less one. As I said before, Manny never got to see the final movie, *Revenge of the Sith*. So of course, when the movie was released, we went to see it. We went to the midnight showing of the movie, which of course was the first showing. We did this because this would have been what he would have done. So we bought the tickets in advance, and we went to see the movie. We sat all in a row, and we left the center seat empty; that was Manny's seat. When the opening credits started and the words "A long time ago, in a galaxy far away" showed on the screen, followed by the words "Star Wars" and the classic theme song started, it brought tears to our eyes. We totally lost it, knowing that he didn't get to see it and knowing how badly he wanted to . . . We all felt that Manny was present. We watched the movie, but it was a bittersweet experience.

Manny was the type that he got the things he wanted the moment it came out, whether it was a video game, game console, movie, or anything else he fancied. I would always ask him why he didn't wait for a sale, why pay full price for them. He always answered that he wanted to get them right away. In retrospect, he did the right thing; it was almost like he knew his time was short, and he wanted to enjoy his prized possession for as long as possible. He always pre-ordered games and bought movie tickets in advance. Many times I would take him to a midnight movie showing or midnight game release. Manny kept a list of things that he wanted and when they were to be released; unfortunately, he never got them. His time just ran out.

Manny loved to walk. It was one of his passions in life, and boy, did he walk quickly. This was a trait he got from his mother. I remember when we lived in Bay Shore and he worked at the Olive Garden in Massapequa, which is a distance of eleven miles. He being who he was, he decided to walk home from Massapequa to Bay Shore. I remember that he was late coming home. We thought that he had to work overtime. When several hours later he arrived, he entered the house and very proudly announced that he had just walked home from his job. I asked him what possessed him to do that. He told us that he wanted to see if he could do it. I don't know how long it took him, but I googled to see how long it would take to walk that distance, and according to them, it would take three hours forty-five minutes. He probably did it in less time, 'cause he walked very fast, much faster than the average person.

Manny was a meticulous person. He always kept his room neat as a pin, again like his mother. All his possessions were kept in a certain place of his choosing. He was very particular of how he kept things. His Star Wars collection was all together over on one side of the room. His video games were in another side, all in order on shelves, and he knew just where each one went. Even his DVDs he kept on shelves, but not on the same shelf as his games; they just didn't go together. I remember when we would want to borrow a movie from him to watch, he would come out to the living room with the movie and place it into the DVD player. Then he would take the controller and start the movie and sit there and watch the movie with us. After the movie ended, he would take the movie out of the player, then he handled the DVD only by the edges and replaced it back into the case. Then he would go back to his room and put it back on the shelf exactly where it was. A bit meticulous, wouldn't you say?

Manny loved holidays; he liked Halloween. He loved getting, as he would say, free candy. He had a saying, "If it's free, it's good for me," and he would say it anytime he would get something for free. He went trick or treating all his life. He was happy he had a younger brother. This way he could go trick or treating. In his later years, he wore his Darth Maul costume, his favorite Star Wars character, and he would take his brother around the neighborhood. People always said, "Wow, you're a big kid," as he would get his treat. Like I said, he was a kid at heart.

He of course loved Christmas, and he would always make a list of things he wanted. His last Christmas he was disappointed that he wasn't working and he couldn't buy gifts. Manny was a giver, and he always got us gifts. Not being able to do so really bothered him. When Christmas morning came, Manny was always the first one out of bed. He would wake up his younger brother and tell him, "Santa Claus came. Let's go see what he brought us." Then like two little elves, they would find their pile of wrapped presents. Then the house would be filled with the sound of paper tearing . . . *Rip!* Then their sounds of "Ooh, look what I got!" Then sounds of laughter. This I remember with joy. Christmas has never been the same in my household. It's like there is a piece missing in the puzzle that is my life.

Manny always had a smile on his face, a smile that I miss dearly. Even though we do put up a tree, albeit a small one, we no longer decorate the outside with lights, and my wife takes the tree down on the day after Christmas.

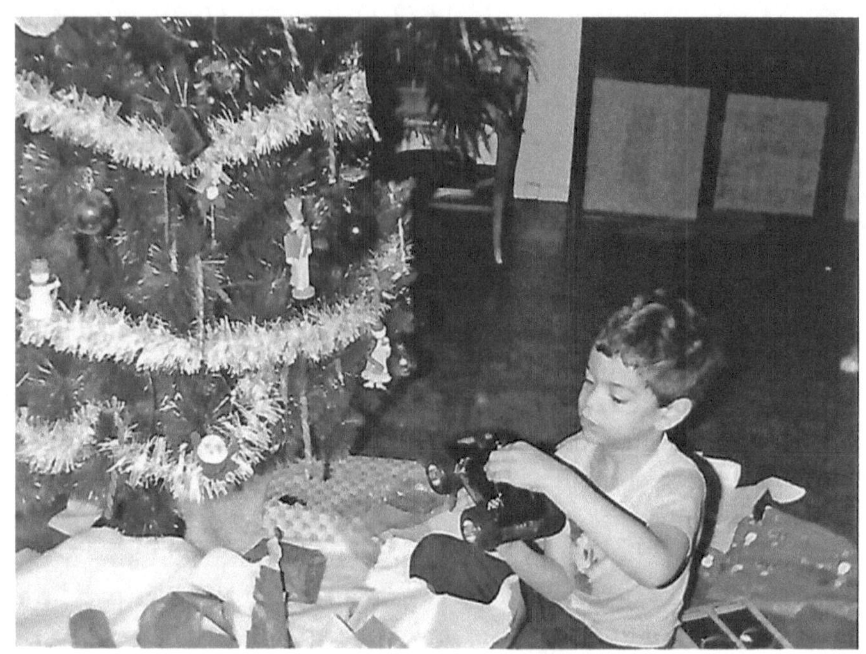

Manny inspecting a new remote control car

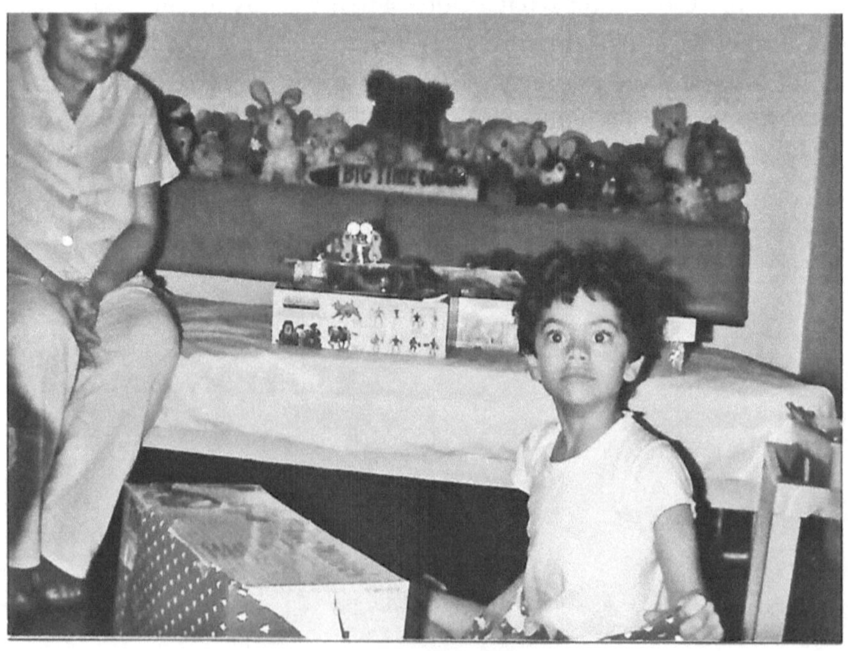

I got what

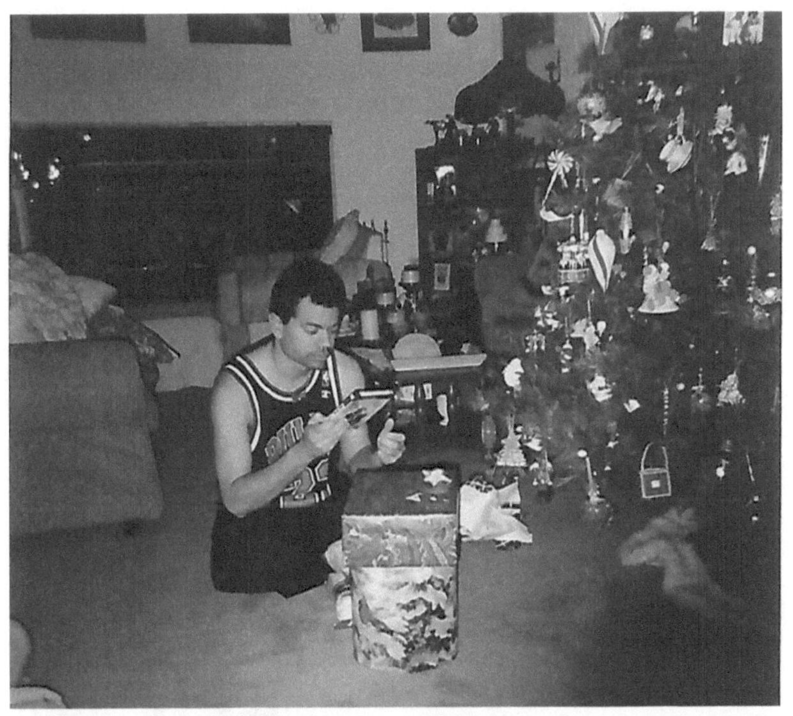

Manny's at Christmas

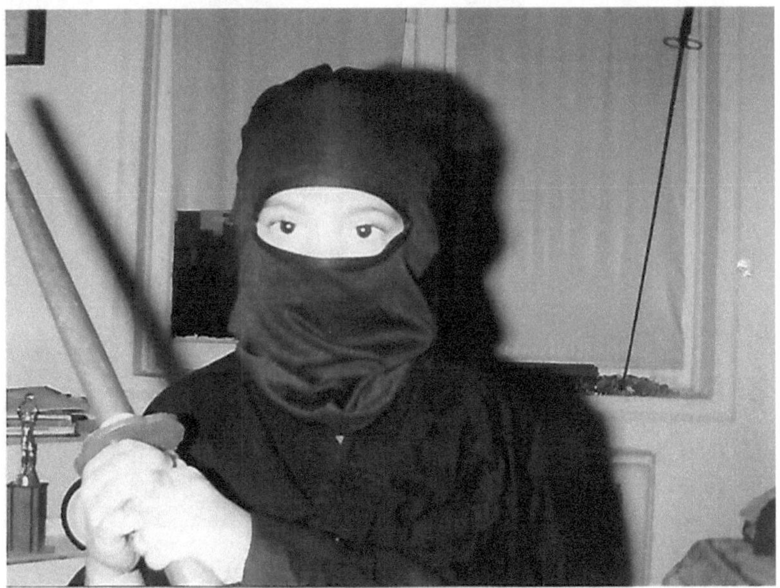

Our little ninja

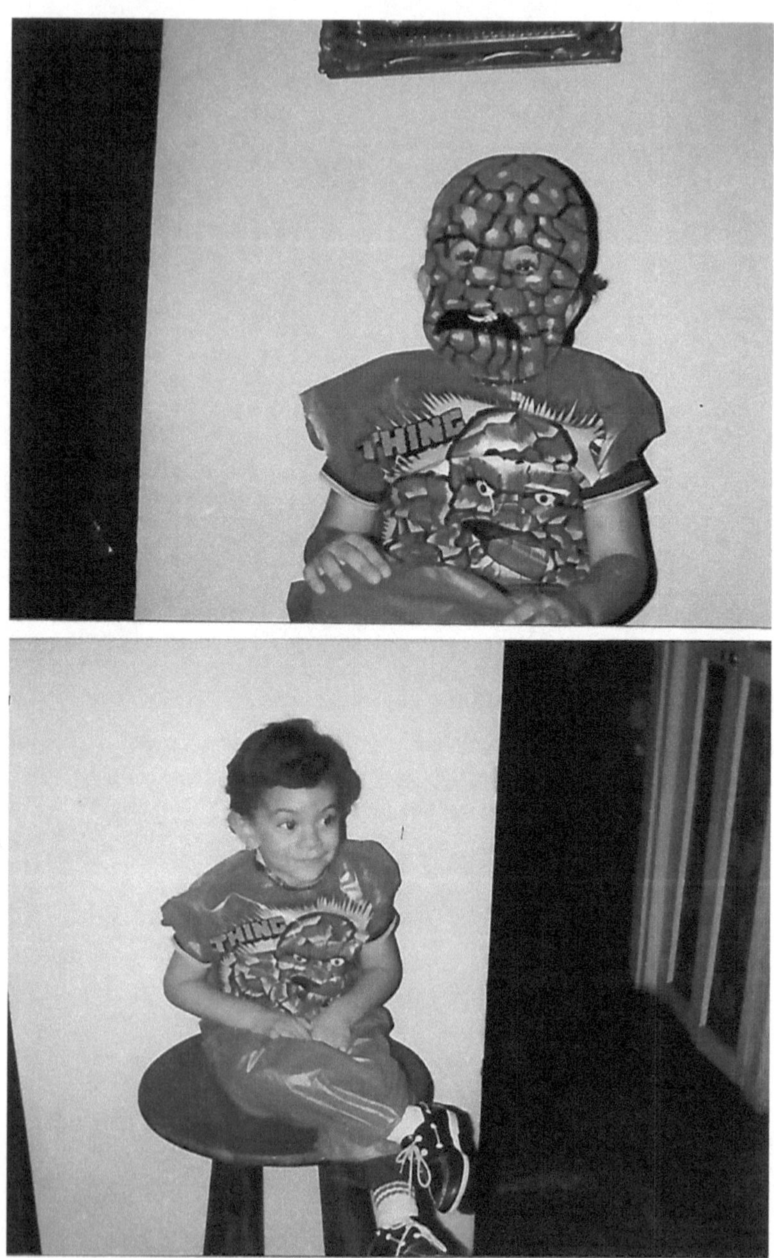

Manny dressed in the Thing costume

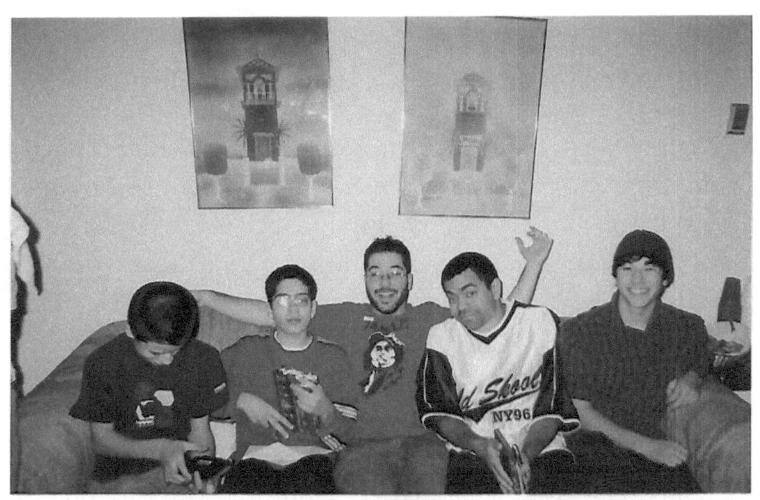

The cousin's last Christmas together

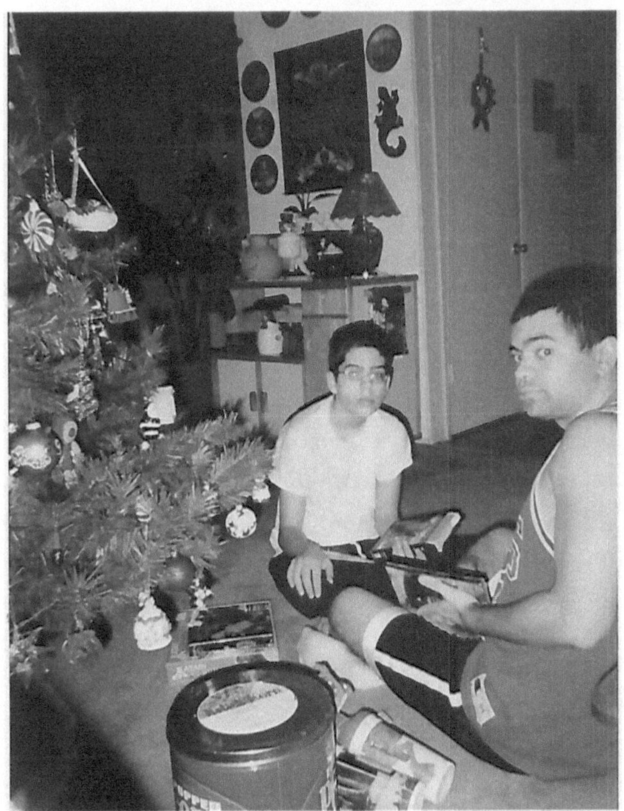

The brothers last Christmas together

Manny always helped people whenever the opportunity arose. I remember one day there was a young man that was trying to catch the train to go home. He needed five dollars to be able to take the train. Manny was going into the local Family Dollar to get some snacks for himself. He told the youth, "Wait here. Let me get what I need, and then I'll help you." Manny made sure he had five dollars left over. When he came out, he found the youth and gave him the last five dollars he had. He left himself broke to help this kid. Not only that, he told him, "My father will take you to the train station, which is about two miles away," which I did. He did this kind of thing often. He liked the feeling of giving; it made him feel good. This was kind of heart that he had, and people loved him for it.

I remember once Pat Benatar, whom my wife is a huge fan of, was coming to Long Island to give a concert. She wanted me to buy tickets so that we could go see her sing. At that particular time, we were experiencing some financial difficulties. I really couldn't afford to buy the tickets for her. I was upset that I couldn't get them for her. Manny, being generous as he always was, bought us the tickets. Needless to say, Levia was so happy that she was going to see the concert. Ironically, Beth Hart opened for her, and her song "I'll Stay with You" was one of the songs that was dedicated to Manny. This was one of many things that Manny did to make another person happy. It was just in his nature to do these kinds of things. He always found a way to do what was right even if he had to sacrifice and not buy something he wanted, just to make someone else happy.

My wife likes to collect the toys that are given by the fast-food places. She has a very extensive collection. Since Manny worked at Wendy's and they too give out toys, she would ask Manny to bring her the toys. She would jokingly tell him, "If you don't bring me the toys, then don't bother coming home."

"Gee, Mom, I have enough to do. Now you want me to remember to bring you toys." He of course would purchase the toys for her. He loved his mom immensely, and he wanted not only to make her happy but also to show her his love for her.

Manny would spend lots of time in his room playing games or watching a movie. When she would want to see him because she hadn't seen him in a while, she would call out his name, "Manny." He of course would answer her call and come to her. Then she would again jokingly say, "Can you pass me this?" She was referring to something, anything that was lying on the coffee table that was actually at arm's length. He would say, "Oh, Mom, you could get that yourself." He would always pick it up and give it to her. She only did this to see his face and his wonderful smile. These were the kind of games that they would play with each other.

Manny mostly worked the closing shift at Wendy's. He used to get home at about 2:00 a.m. or so. When he had something to tell his mother, of course he couldn't wait. He would stand at the bottom of the stairs and say, "Mom, are you up?" She of course would get up, and they would talk about whatever he couldn't wait to tell her. Sometimes after being home for a while and he wanted a snack, he would go to the kitchen. He would make popcorn, and we would be awakened by the popping sound of the popcorn in the microwave oven. These are some of things that made Manny . . . Manny. How we miss these things.

Manny used to love fish sticks; he always did even as a child. He especially loved to make fish stick sandwiches. He loved to pile up the fish, putting ten or twelve sticks per sandwich. I would tell him that he didn't need to put so many sticks in the sandwiches. I foolishly complained that I was buying so many bags of fish sticks. Now in hindsight, if I knew his days were numbered, I would have never complained about him eating so many sticks. I would have told him, "Manny, eat as many sticks as you want. Don't worry, I'll get more." How foolish I was worrying about something as trivial as fish sticks.

Manny had gotten a surround sound system for his room. He had all his gaming consoles, his TV, and his stereo connected to it. Of course, when you have a surround sound, you want to enjoy it, and he of course did. Since he was sort of a night owl because he worked late, he would use it late at night while we were sleeping. When he would play his games, we would be startled from a sound sleep, hearing loud booms from the games. I would tell him to lower it, we couldn't sleep. This would sort of annoy him. In reality, when you went to his room, he really didn't have it that loud, but the sounds would travel through the wall, and it actually sounded louder upstairs in our room than it sounded in his room. It was just the nature of the surround sound. He would either lower it further or put on headphones. These little things bothered us when he was alive. Now that he has passed, I got to tell you I miss them terribly. What I wouldn't do to hear those booms of the surround sound. These are stupid things that bothered us at that time and now we miss. So don't ever let things bother you in life, because you are going to miss them in death, trust me.

Manny did not like to get me upset, so he did his best to prevent this from happening. When my wife would see something on one of the shopping networks, he would always tell her, "Don't get it. You don't want to upset Dad." If she insisted on getting it, he would buy it for her. This way I wouldn't get upset. He was always doing things like that to prevent me from getting mad. He wanted to keep the peace. This is something that he did because of the love and admiration he had for me. I miss him.

Manny one day bought a movie called *Pitch Black* for his mother. This was a movie she wanted to own, and he knew it. So he went out and got it for her. Manny had already gotten sick by this time, but he spent the last of his money and used it to make his mother happy. Every day in the months that my wife would spend trying desperately to save her son's life, he would ask her, "Mom, did you see the movie yet?"

She answered him, "Not yet, Manny. I've been so busy lately, but don't worry. I'll watch it."

"Okay, Mom, don't but forget to see the movie."

"I will," she said. This was a constant thing that happened on a daily basis. Unfortunately, she never saw the movie while he was alive.

Then finally after two years, which was the time we didn't watch TV because of our grief, she finally went to watch the movie, and lo and behold, she found a note that he had placed inside the case. The note read as follows:

> To Mom, Thanks for all u have done in the past, present and the future. I will always be yours and u will always be my #1 lady. Love Manny L.

My wife cried and cried. She was distraught the entire day. Now she understood why he kept asking her if she had seen the movie. He wanted her to find this little message of his love for her. I know that you have no way of knowing this, but as I just wrote this chapter, I had to pause because I started crying. After all this time, eleven years, Manny is still touching my heart with his love that he had for us. Manny, we miss you so much!

Manny also liked the animated show *Futurama*. I can still hear him laugh as he would watch it. After he died, we would watch all the seasons that he owned over and over. This kind of made us feel like he was still with us. It was a way that we dealt with our grief over our loss. We did this in the two years that we didn't watch cable TV. We did this not only in his honor but also for personal reasons. We would at first watch this show with tear-filled eyes. We were in a constant state of tears. Eventually, we were able to watch them and enjoy them just as he did. Manny always wanted us to watch it together, and we really never did. I foolishly took it for granted that there was always tomorrow, but tomorrow never came. We ran out of tomorrows. So take it from me all of you who are reading this. Don't take things for granted, spend time with your children, and do things together. Don't save things for tomorrow, because tomorrow may never come. Live in the now, because it can be taken away in the blink of an eye.

I love the Lord of the Rings movies. I wanted to watch them with Manny, and he didn't want to see them with me as each movie came out because he wanted to watch them all together. He knew that there was going to be three movies made, and he didn't want to wait for the next one to come out. He hated cliffhangers. He was already waiting for the Star Wars finale, and he hated waiting. We didn't go to the movies much. We mostly wait for the videos to come out. The last of these movies was released on video in 2004, the year that he got sick. Needless to say, we never watched them together, unfortunately. I know he would have loved them.

My wife also started listening to his music after his passing. She never really cared for it when he was alive. I too didn't care for it much. While my wife listened, I would listen to the songs also.

I got say that both of us "now" like his music. We like Metallica, Godsmack, Linkin Park, and others that he would listen to. There was one song that Manny dedicated to "death," only because he was facing that possibility, not because he wanted die. On the contrary, he wanted to live. He played it to his mom, and one part in particular is the reason why he dedicated it to "death." The title of the song is "I Am" by Godsmack. The part of the lyrics said, "Death can wait till I'm good and ready."

I am an avid Star Trek fan, and Manny would tape the shows that aired on TV for me because I was working. He taped the *Next Generation* and *Deep Space Nine* for me. No matter what, he never missed an episode. He always made sure he was home so that he could tape them for me. Then he would watch the episodes with me even though he had already seen it. Thanks, Manny, for being you.

When Manny got sick, he never let that take the joy out his life. He always expected the best of all situations. He faced his sickness like a man. He never complained about it; he never said, "Woe is me." He faced death like a warrior, something I hope when my time comes I will be able to do. Manny was very brave, and he will forever be my hero. I learned how to face adversity with my head held high. I thank him for that, and even though he had the heart of a kid, he matured with this horrifying experience he was facing. It just made him have a stronger character and hold his head high. This made me a better person, and I learned that from him. I hope I make him as proud of me as he made me proud of him. After all, he was a hard act to follow.

Manny had a girlfriend that he had just started dating. She is a beautiful young woman, and she kind of reminds me of Levia. We were to meet her while he was alive, but we never did. We did meet her after his death. I don't really know why we never met her while he was alive. But I do remember him telling Levia, "Mom, wait till you meet my girlfriend. You're going to love her." I figure he didn't want her to see him sick. And eleven years since his death, she leaves him one red and one black carnation, representing his favorite colors, on his birthday and anniversary of his death without fail. I think this was the one for Manny; she would have been my daughter-in-law.

Manny kept journals, and he would constantly write things in them. We knew he kept a journal, but of course, we never read it until after he passed. This was his last journal after he got sick. I would like to share some of it with you. This way you can see the way he thought and who he was. I know he would want me to share it. On the inside of the front cover, there is a picture of him holding his gizmo stuffy, which he cherished; and over the picture, he wrote, "To my family and friends." These are the highlights of what he wrote:

> There's a difference between knowing the path . . . and walking the path. To hell with opportunity. I create opportunity. I want to die the way I live. Try not, do or do not, there is no try. All knowledge ultimately means self-knowledge. Use your brain to overcome your enemy. Do not seek for it for it will come when least expected. The highest art is no art. The highest form is no form. ML.

> In a world gone bad I try to show goodness! What makes you happy in life is what is most important. I am not scared of life, it should be scared of me! I try to do my best, therefore I am the best. I rather die on my feet than live on my knees!! We do not live for . . . we simply live. There is no help but self help. Using no way as way, having no limitation as limitation. I am, therefore I Know I am!! To break a fear, U must face it! Most important thing is that life is fun!! I believe in myself, that's all I need! I learn to fight for what I believe and I will!! That which does not kill us makes us stronger. The key to immortality is first living a life worth remembering. ML.

> I always knew my life was going to be different. I had fun throughout my life. And that is what is most important, I think. I did not want to be

just another bad person in this world. People that meant a lot in my life friends, family, but there are people that are close to me. One of them that I always loved, Bruce Lee. Yes he is the greatest martial artist. He did not stop living for no one and I love that. Also I love Michael Jordan, he meant a lot in my life. I learned a lot from these guys. I was always at peace when walking and playing video games. I did not want to be just another bad guy, so I did the other way, to be good. ML.

I am without a doubt my mother, strong and hard headed, Ha! Ha! It's like something inside is telling me to work out and go about yourself. Maybe it's a guy I love a lot . . . Bruce Lee he did not stop for no one, sort of like me. I choose to live, that's very important to me. ML.

Let's talk about something that's been all my life . . . STAR WARS. It's more than just a bunch of space movies. I grew up with and will die with it. I always wanted to be a Jedi and I feel that I am in this life. I learned to be good and to trust my feelings about this world. The one person who started this love is my uncle Jr when I was little. I am watching right now ha ha, Return of the Jedi. I can't wait for the last one. I thank George Lucas for putting something good in my life. Manny L.

I like the Matrix so much because I felt like Neo. When I was born, there was something different about my life and was going have to fight for what I knew in my heart to be right and not wrong. That's why I like Bruce Lee, he did what he wanted and let no one tell him different. ML.

Another thing video games or walking are not the only things that I am at peace with. I did love playing sports, volleyball, hockey, soccer (goalie) but most of all basketball. I love playing and I think I could do my best, thinking and I am free. I can't wait to play it again. I am happy to have true friends in my life and I hope to have more. ML.

With all this stuff going on. My heart and all I learned in life. I learned to be good and try to teach what I believe in my heart. That's why I have so much to do. If my other family wants to see me, that's ok I forgive. I'll tell them I have a true family and my friends are also a part of me. ML.

The following are taken from other journals he kept throughout his life. He did them for school. These are just a few excerpts:

9/27/96. I can't wait for Halloween. I am going to go all over Long Island. I am going to get a ton of candy. Most of all I will hang out with my friends. I am looking forward to it! I love holidays, it is a great time to have fun. This weekend I will be making money, which is good! Because I am trying to save as much as I can. Thanks for reading. ML.

9/30/96. I love Florida, it has great weather. My favorite ride in MGM Studios in Orlando would have to be The Tower of Terror. You go through a hotel that is about 20 stories. Then they drop you 13 stories from an elevator it was great!! When I was in Florida this summer I stayed in a cool hotel, with a huge pool. My favorite ride in Disney World would have to be Space Mountain, it was very fast! When you get inside it looks like you are in space. It is a rollercoaster ride. Universal Studio was my favorite place of all. They had T2 in 3D, when you get inside they give you 3D glasses. It's like a 3D movie but it makes it look like you are in it. I also went on Jaws the ride. Jaws attacks the boat while you are in it!! They also had a ride called Kongfrontation, King Kong attacks a train. I also went on Back to the Future the ride, well it's not a ride you go into a car with a big screen in front of you the screen and seats move, so it makes you feel like a ride and that you are in the movie Florida is a great place to visit! Don't miss Disney World, Magic Kingdom, Epcot, MGM Studio and my favorite Universal Studios. ML.

12/2/96. I wanted to write about how people judge others. I think people should not just look at the outside person but the inside person. That's what counts the most in life. This is a subject I've see a lot of. It hurts when a person or one of my friends gets picked on by the way they dress or how they look. You can have a person that dresses all cool and that is a mean person. It should be that looks don't count at all. The only time looks should count is when you are going for a job and the interviewer sees you dress sloppy. See people judge on looks and what's in your head. See family does not judge you on how you look. When I went to my aunt's house for thanksgiving when I sat down they don't judge on how you dress or look. That's why I like family than other people. Sometimes people can be mean and cold hearted. But there are a lot of nice people that care in this world. And that's the best people on this earth other than family. ML.

12/16/97. My thoughts on fear. Fear can be a bad thing. When a person has fear he/she is scared of something. Maybe he/she does not understand that thing. I don't recall having any fears or anything like that. I think that when you grow up most of the fears you had as a child go away. When you were a child sometimes it was maybe that you were afraid of the dark. Now in my life maybe not fitting in school can be a kind of a fear. But when you look fear in the eyes you can accomplish anything. As I am writing this it reminds me of those t-shirts that have that saying about what I am writing about. Can you guess what it is . . . NO FEAR! ML.

[Not dated.] Now that I am twenty one, I realized that in the past few years my relationship with my parents has changed. I am more mature now that I have grown up. My parents trust me more now than when I was a teenager. I help around the house and work part time. My other responsibility is going to school at night. My parents appreciate how I help around the house. We have more in common now that we share responsibilities. Now we look at life in the same way. We all work to pay bills, while sharing in the care of the house. My parents are proud of my accomplishments. I had a good childhood, as I was growing up my parents were there to help me. And because they were supportive I did well in high school. My parents look back at my childhood with fond memories. My parents are proud of themselves for doing a great job bringing up their son. ML

[Not dated.] They got me out of trouble. My parents helped me learned to take responsibilities in life. My parents showed me how to get a job and how to support myself in life. ML.

As you can see, Manny was a kid at heart. But he did have some interesting, if not admirable, philosophies. But one thing is for sure: he wanted to do good and be good, and he did and he was. He also never wanted to judge people unfairly, and he didn't. He always tried to find a silver lining in every dark storm cloud. I do know that it bothered him that he had gotten sick. It put a dampener on the way he lived. He didn't walk as much, not because he didn't want to, but because we were afraid he might suffer a seizure. This was hard for him, because as you read, it made him feel free.

We didn't want him to work so he couldn't earn his money and go be with his friends. We did allow him to work for a while, but we were afraid that something would happen to him. So we asked him to stop working, and him always wanting to please us, he stopped working. So he spent his time mostly with his brother, playing video games. He watched his favorite movies, and he made the best out of a bad situation. He also witnessed his mom trying desperately to get him taken care of. I'm sure that was hard on him even though he didn't say anything. I can only imagine the pain and anguish that he must've felt. He was the type to help people, and now when he needed help, no one would help him.

Manny didn't have any enemies. I know this may sound unusual, but it was true. Like I said before, he never judged people. He would accept people and see the good in them. He wasn't prejudice; he didn't care about ethnic backgrounds, religions, creeds, or age. He saw the good in everyone and everything. He was an old soul. Manny was the kindest individual I ever knew. He would give you the shirt right off his back. He was like a child experiencing things for the first time; he was in awe of everything. He lived life in the moment, in the now. I learned many things from Manny. I am glad that I had the privilege to have had him in my life, to call him my son and especially him calling me dad. I will never forget him, and I miss him so much. He made life extra special. Thank you, Manny, for all you were and for showing me what's important in life. May you always rest in peace! This is a very brief history of what and who he was, and words cannot truly show how special he was. I pray you can at least see just how truly exceptional he was.

We believe Manny was our angel. We used to see life through rose-colored glasses. We were never concerned with the way the world was changing for the worse. We weren't concerned with the injustices around us. We, like him, only saw the good. When he passed on, those rose-colored glasses were ripped off our eyes. We now saw how ugly the world was becoming. We saw the injustices; we saw how the world had lost its morals. We started seeing how when we held the door for someone as we entered a mall or store, how many people didn't say thank you. I started noticing how other people were not courteous when driving. We saw how people were becoming selfish; we were becoming a "me" generation. Many people would not help another person unless there was something in it for them. We started seeing how children were disrespecting their parents. Levia and I were not raised this way, and we didn't raise our children this way.

Well, now I'm going to pick up where I left off. We buried Manny, and we left him in the earth, gone but never forgotten, ever. We were numb from the whole experience. We swore that we would make sure he didn't die in vain. We didn't want any parent to go through what we went through. In fact, we didn't want anyone else to go through it, whether it is a child, parent, friend, spouse, etc. We live in the USA, and it is inexcusable that this can happen here.

Have we become a society where money is more important than a person's life? God, I hope not. But this shows that not everything should be left to the private sector. There are things that are more precious than money, and life is one of them. We need universal health care in this country. The sooner Americans wake up and realize this, the sooner we can fix our broken health-care system. We have to stop listening to politicians about how our system shouldn't change. They are a bunch of hypocrites that have a Cadillac health-care insurance for life. That we pay for, by the way.

I have spoken to people about these facts. Most people believe that we don't have the power to change things. I am tired of hearing, "Yeah, but what are we going to do?" Like our voices don't matter. Now imagine if when our nation's founders had this attitude. When Paul Revere got on his horse to announce that the Red Coats are coming. Imagine if the people opened their windows and doors and said, "Yeah, well, what are you going to do?" Where would we be as a nation? We wouldn't be one that's where we would be. We as the people can make a difference.

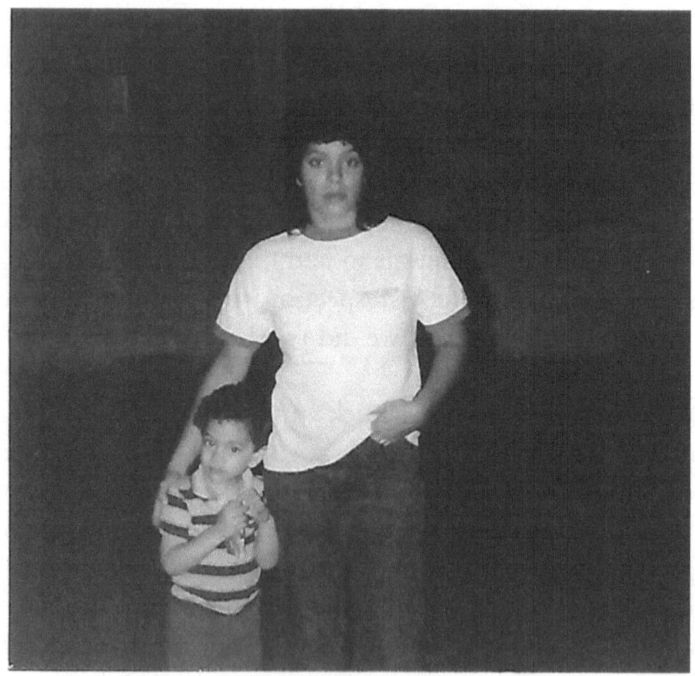

Mother and Son

Manny had a unique laugh; I can still hear it in my mind. His laugh would bring you so much joy that even if you were sad, it would make you laugh also. I can't really remember Manny not smiling or laughing about something. I remember him once telling me a story about a friend of his. He had gone to Great Adventure with his friends. His friend had tripped on something, but when they saw that there was nothing that could have made him trip, he asked his friend, "What did you trip on?" His friend answered, "I tripped on air." Manny would burst out into laughter while he was telling the story. I still remember it vividly with fond memories.

Losing Manny took its toll on the entire family. We never in our wildest dreams imagined that Manny was going to die. Like I said earlier, I have a friend that had an AVM. His condition wasn't curable either. He was treated for his condition, and he is alive and living a normal life. He does have to take an antiseizure medicine and has to take it for the rest of his life. My friend was given a chance to live by his doctors. Manny was not given this chance. He didn't fall through the cracks; he was shoved into the cracks, and he was stepped on like he was a nobody. How Levia and I never lost our cool is only because of our faith in God. He gave us the strength to go through what had happened and what was yet to come.

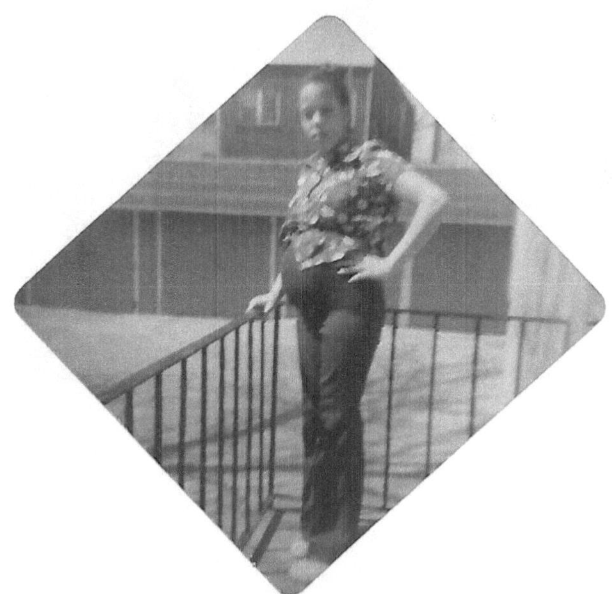

Levia carrying Manny in her belly

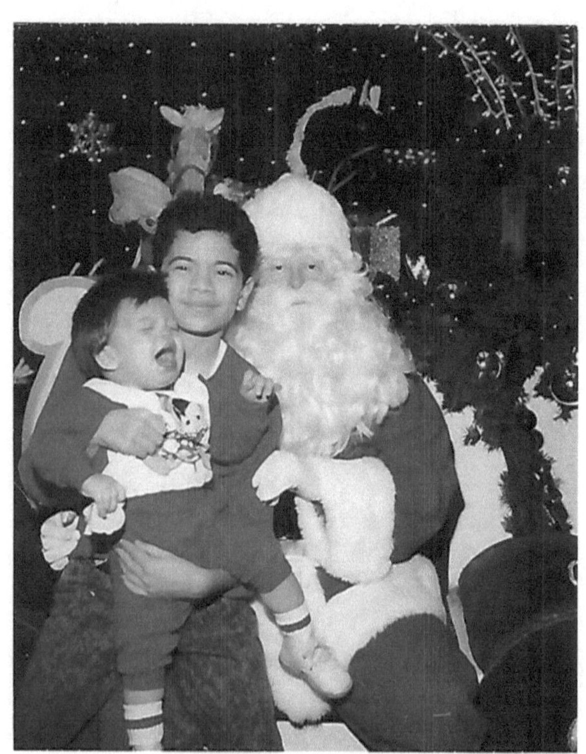

AHH Santa is a monster

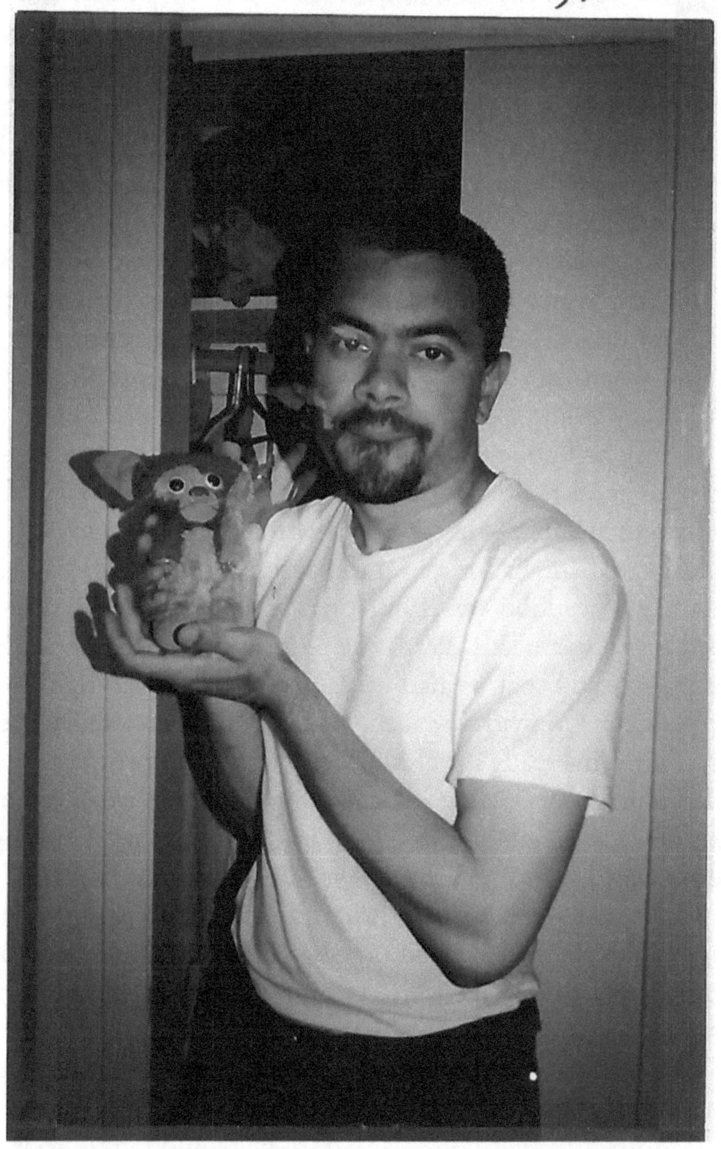


Manny holding Gizmo for the last time he wrote to my family and friends
He was sick and his hand writing was shaky at this point he was degrading
This was on the inside cover of his last journal
and gizmo was buried with him

So we decided to get Manny's hospital records before anything went missing. We didn't tell the doctors or hospitals that Manny had died yet. So we got his records, and we started to sift through them. I was appalled to see how the lack of insurance was indeed an issue as to why Manny was neglected. I found a record from Dr. Niimi and Berenstein's office stating, as per Dr. Niimi, when patient's insurance (Medicaid) was in place, he would be taken care of. Appalling! Others stated that patient's care may be restricted due to lack of insurance. It was heartbreaking to say the least.

Then we decided to sue, and we went to see an attorney. We went to a law office in Babylon, New York. I won't mention their names because I don't want to waste the ink. They know who they are if and when they are reading this. We told them our story, and they said they would take the case. They were outraged to hear about what Manny had gone through. We were under the impression that we were in good hands. Well, as it turned out, we weren't. We got called into their office—my wife, my younger son, and myself. Then she told us that she had received the autopsy result and that Manny did not die of a blood vessel bursting, which is what we suspected. He died as a result of his AVM; she bluntly stated that he was going to die anyway and that we had no case. She stated that right in front of my younger son who was already heartbroken and angry over this whole affair. This really upset him, and with good reason.

I couldn't believe what I was hearing. How can we have no case? He was neglected. She told us that it didn't matter since he was going to die anyway. I still can't believe that this—I want to use the *C* word here, but I won't—this woman just said that. She actually wanted us to forget about it, that we had no case. This was something that we were not going to do. We weren't going to take no for an answer. I told her in not so many words that wasn't happening. She then told us to wait as she went and got the senior partner. He came out and tried to say the same thing. Then he said he would see if we had any other recourse and that if we wanted to, he would look into it. I was furious, and I told him, "I don't want you doing a damn thing," and I fired them on the spot. My son and I stormed out of the office. I first thought about taking his file that was within arm's length, but I didn't. So now we didn't have an attorney.

We decided to get another attorney, and I got to say that was easier said than done. We saw attorney after attorney; we went to see six others. All of them showed some interest, but ultimately they all declined the case. One of them had told us, "Do you expect me to spend money and time to get back little for my work?"

How can this be? I thought. There has to be someone that would help us. Ten months after his death and still no attorney. We were getting concerned because there is a two-year time limit to file a lawsuit, and time was ticking away.

Then in February 2005, we decided to make an official complaint against the hospital and the doctors. We sent our complaint of the hospital to the State of New York Department of Health. The complaint of the doctors was sent to the Office of Professional Medical Conduct, which is a department of the Department of Health. We sent a brief story of what happened to Manny, along with specific areas we wanted addressed. We got a letter of acknowledgment that they received the complaint. But by June 8, the case was closed. The letter we received said that Manny had an inoperable tumor and that any delays wouldn't have made a difference in the outcome. They swept the problem under the table. They weren't even smart enough to get his condition correct. Manny had a treatable AVM, not an inoperable tumor. This is the reason that doctors cannot discipline doctors. They just won't go against each other. We were shocked but, to tell you the truth, not at all surprised. But we decided to press on. Bureaucracy and corruption would not defeat us. Hey, when God is with us, who can be against us?

We decided to tell the media. We called the New York TV networks, and we got no response. We tried some of the local papers and still nothing. We tried and tried, and we seemed to be hitting brick walls. No one, it seemed, was interested in his story. So here we were, frustrated that we didn't have an attorney. Now we faced the possibility that we couldn't get his story told. It seemed every avenue we pursued, the road would lead to nowhere. But we were persistent, and where there is a will, there is a way. We kept trying to get his story told. We would not take no for an answer. This was a very stressful time for us, but persistence pays.

We tried to get some politicians involved. We contacted local officials, such as Tim Foley, who was Suffolk County executive; we got no response from him. Then we went to the state level, such as Senator Trunzo and Elliot Spitzer, who was state attorney general at that time. They didn't even respond to our queries. We then decided to try the federal level. Our congressional representative Tim Bishop did acknowledge us. In fact, we met with him on several occasions. He was compassionate and understanding to our situation, but his ability to help us was limited.

So then we decided to start a petition and called it Justice for Manny. We were going stand in front of grocery stores, malls, libraries, and anywhere we could think of to get signatures. We were going to send it to our United States senators in Washington, DC, that represent New York State. We were requesting a Senate investigation surrounding the circumstances of Manny. We figured if the Senate can investigate baseball and the use of steroids, which seems to be a trivial matter, they would be able to investigate what we believe was a matter of much more importance. The petition read as follows:

> Dear Mr. Chuck Schumer and Mrs. Hillary Rodham-Clinton:
>
> We the People of New York State are outraged at the injustice that has happened to Manuel N. Lanza Jr. This young man lost his life because of a "glitch" in our healthcare system. How can this happen in the United States of America? We are a world superpower, the so-called "policeman" of the world. We now have a matter that affects all Americans, and we need a "policeman" to investigate this serious situation. We cannot leave this to other doctors because it causes a conflict of interest. We cannot leave this to lawyers

because they are only in it for the money, not for the injustice or to make things right.

Here we have a twenty-four-year-old man named Manuel N. Lanza Jr. A young man loved by his community. A hardworking young man who loved life. A courteous and helpful young man who didn't deserve the lack of care that he got for a serious condition. A young man who wasn't a drug user or a troublemaker. A young man that was never sick before in his life. Then when he is diagnosed with a serious condition, he is denied the proper care because of lack of insurance. This is inexcusable! Something must be done about this so that this can never happen again to any American. This man had a "right" to receive the proper treatment, a "right" that was revoked because of greed.

He was sent to the supposed top doctors in their field, and because of greed, his treatment was delayed and delayed until it cost him his life. The legal system doesn't work either because:

    a) Doctors do not want to go against their own, especially when the doctor involved is the top in the field. Even if a New York State medical examiner says the doctors were negligent. This doesn't matter because the malpractice laws require you to have another physician in the same field go against the other. These guys work with each other and rely on each other in the field. This causes of conflict of interest.

    b) Because he was unmarried with no children, the money that can be recovered is limited because it is the parents that are suing. Lawyers, once they realize this and that there is little money involved, don't want anything to do with the case. Even though they are outraged, so justice cannot be served. This makes doctors "above the law" and no one is above the law.

So in light of these events we are signing this petition and are asking for a Senate investigation surrounding the circumstances of Manuel N. Lanza Jr.'s death. Please be our policeman and please see to it that the parties involved are held accountable. Don't let this injustice go unpunished. Everyone is entitled to due process in this country. Please see that Manuel gets his due process. We want Justice for Manny.

This was signed by hundreds of individuals.

After this we received a letter from Mrs. Clinton dated August 8, 2005. It reads as follows:

Dear Mrs. Prieto:

Thank you for your correspondence dated June 15, 2005 regarding your healthcare matter.

In an effort to further assist you, I have contacted the Office of Patient Relations at St. Luke's-Roosevelt Hospital Center and have asked for a review of the information of the information you have presented. I will be in touch with you when the agency response is received.

Please be assured I will continue to do everything possible to help you in this matter.

Sincerely yours,<br>
Signed Hillary Rodham Clinton

She also sent us a copy of the letter she sent to the director of patient relations at St. Luke's. It basically said to investigate the situation and to let her know the outcome.

There was never a senate investigation made. Most likely because of the events that followed, which I will tell in detail. Mrs. Clinton, however, is a proponent for universal health care here in the United States. I am also a believer in universal care. Now that she is running for president, I hope that if she wins, she keeps her campaign promise to push for universal health care. This would definitely stop this type of situation from happening again. Let's us wait and see.

Then one day I brought the *New York Post* home from work. My wife didn't look at it at first, but the next day, while I was at work, she did. She was angry because on the front page was a silly story about two girls hiring a bouncer because they were tired of being hit on when they went out. Outraged, she called the *Post* and told them that she couldn't believe the story they put on their front page. She told them, "Let me tell you about what happened to my son." She told them the story, and she was connected to a reporter. Her name is Susan Edelman, and she immediately wanted to print Manny's story.

Sue (the name she told us to call her) came to our house with a photographer, and we went through everything. We showed her records and proof of our story. She gathered all she needed. We were photographed, and she told us, "I will print his story." God bless her; she did. The *Post* decided to print his story in the Sunday edition. She only asked that we give her the exclusive to the story, which we agreed to. She graciously sent us a copy of the story the day before, which was Saturday. We were emotional. Manny's story was going to finally be told. We read and loved the story, and we approved its context.

So on Sunday, November 27, 2005, the story broke. There it was, printed in a major New York newspaper for all to see. "Left To Die," read the headlines. "Hosp said no insurance, no surgery." And there was a picture of my wife, along with Manny's picture.

> EXCLUSIVE An anguished mother says her 24-year-old son died waiting for brain surgery at an elite Manhattan hospital because he had no health

insurance. "When you get insurance, we'll take care of your son," Levia Prieto says a hospital administrator at St. Luke's Roosevelt Hospital Center told her repeatedly in the months before she found her son, Manny Lanza, dead in his bedroom. Federal and state "patient dumping" laws forbid hospitals from denying emergency care based on lack of insurance. Full Story: pages 4 & 5.

We were ecstatic at his story finally being told. This set off a series of events that opened up a Pandora's box. Our prayers were answered.

In that same edition, there was another story about the health commissioner; Dr. Antonia Novella had ordered a full investigation of Manny's death and a probe of the Health Department's "inexcusable error" in handling our complaints. This was done because of questions raised by the *Post*. They were "busted," and they knew it. They tried to sweep it under the rug, but now the story went public. She was trying to save face. In the article it said she had called my wife, but in reality, she called the next day that the article had come out. My wife says she was a very insincere and cold. She was just trying to save herself. I'm sure she was in hot water. She told my wife that she was outraged about their "inexcusable error" and that she was reopening every aspect of the case. She was a phony; she was just trying to make herself look good. In my opinion, she was just a person put in a position that was more than she could handle. A wannabe!

Sue called us later in the day and asked us if it was okay to give out our phone number to other media sources and to Christine Quinn, who was the newly elected speaker of the New York City Council. We told her that it was all right. We wanted Manny's story to be told; we thought the more the merrier. Then like a big flood, the phone calls started. We got calls from all the major networks, along with other newspapers, all except our local newspaper, *Newsday*, and our local news, News 12 Long Island.

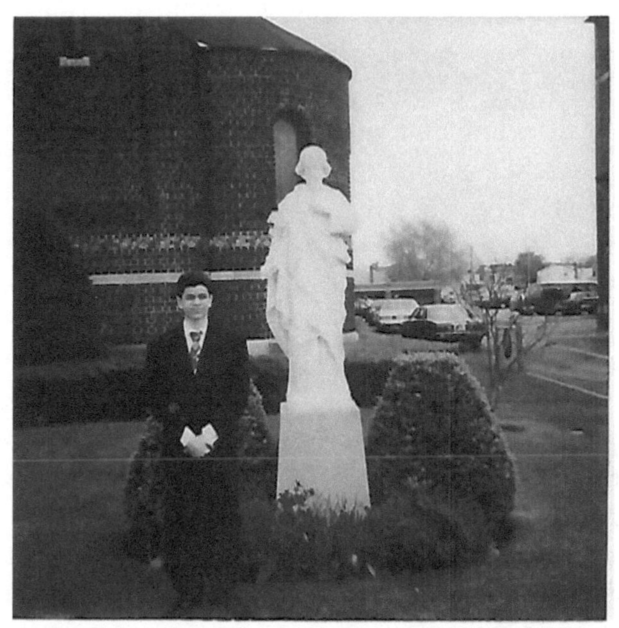

Manny's First Holy Communion in Babylon Long Island

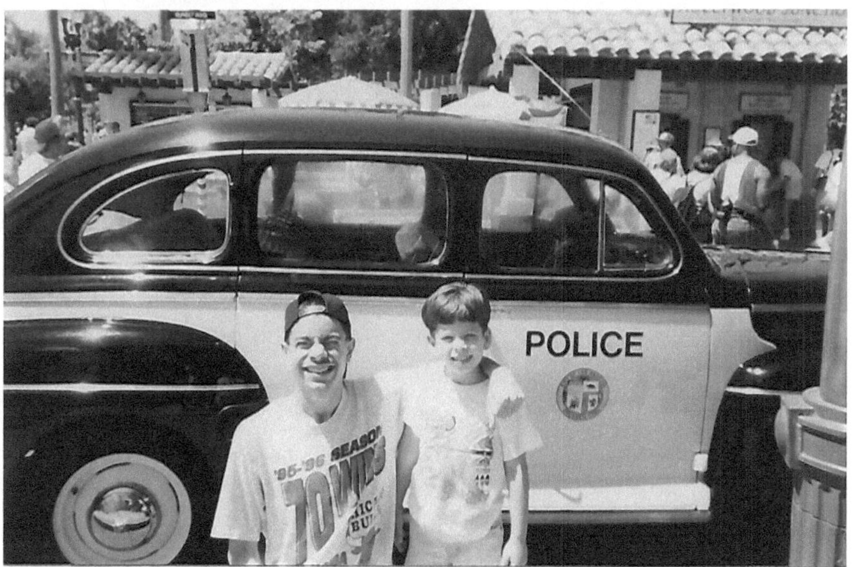


The Brothers at Universal Studios in Florida

All the news stations including the Latin ones wanted interviews, and we agreed to every one of them. Then one by one we were interviewed by every major network, including the Spanish ones. We spent about twelve hours giving interviews, one right behind the other. We were telling his tragic story over and over. Each and every time we cried while making the news crew cry; it was such an emotional story. His story was being told all over the television. We were overwhelmed. We were happy that the world was hearing the horror that we went through that ultimately claimed Manny's life.

Then another prayer was answered, one we didn't expect. Our doorbell rang, and there standing on our porch was an attorney. His name is Mitch Carlinsky. Several days earlier, I told my boss we were having a problem hiring an attorney. He told me that he knew of an attorney that might be able help us. I had no idea that he had talked to him and given him my address. So while we were being interviewed and the press was waiting on line in my driveway and in the street, waiting for their turn for an interview, Mitch was at my door to see if he could help us.

He came in, and we told him our story. He told us that he would try to help us, so we hired him right then and there. The interviews continued, then we got a call from Christine Quinn, the newly elected speaker of the New York City Council. She wanted to talk to Levia concerning passing a law to prevent this from happening again. My wife was happy with the prospects of the law, as was I. Levia was told that her staff would call us to set a date to meet with her in NYC town hall. Through the chaos of the news crews, she calmed my wife down; she was a voice of reason. We finished off the interviews, and even though we stopped watching TV, we watched all the news broadcast, watching Manny's story unfold.

The next day Sue again called us and told us that there was a follow-up story in the *Post*. I immediately went out to buy a copy of the *Post*. We were overwhelmed with emotions when we read the newspaper. Right there in the front page again was a picture of Manny. In big bold letters, the headline read, Manny's Law. Then underneath in smaller but bold underlined letters was "Angry pols vow to end hosp horror." Then under that in regular print read the following:

> Lawmakers are pushing to enact "Manny's Law"—legislation that could prevent the kind of tragedy that led to the death of Manuel Lanza (left), whose family says was denied a lifesaving operation because he had no health insurance. SEE PAGE 5.

We were ecstatic. Not only was his story told, but now our prayers were answered again. Manny would not have died in vain. I got goose bumps; Manny had always said to us, "I will live forever." I always told him that no one lives forever; everyone dies. Manny's words stood out in my mind, and then here I see Manny's Law. Manny in essence was going to live forever. He was going to have a law named after him. We called Sue back and thanked her for the follow-up story. Sue thanked us for the privilege of telling Manny's story to the world. Susan Edelman will always have a special place in our hearts. Thank you, Sue, for being a compassionate person and for all you've done to help us in a very trying time for my family. We will never forget you.

Christine Quinn's office called us, and we set up an appointment to see her. We were excited about getting a law passed. We didn't want the horror that happened to Manny happen to anyone again. Enough is enough! Our health-care system is broken, and we were determined to get it fixed. How dare these doctors and this hospital play God and decide who lives and who dies? Their job is to care of the sick regardless of circumstances, in Manny's case, not having health insurance. But because of greed, they chose that Manny's life wasn't worth saving. As we found out later, there are funds available for cases like Manny's. The state has millions of dollars available just for cases like these, and the doctors and the hospital knew this. They never told us about these funds, and we had no idea that they existed. This should be a criminal act, and the doctors especially should be stripped of their license, forever banned from practicing medicine again. I'm sure if this were the law, this would never happen to anyone, but alas, it's not. Anyway, we set a date to meet with Christine Quinn, and we were eager to meet her.

The day came for us to meet with Christine Quinn. We asked our attorney, Mitch, to accompany us, and he agreed. When we arrived at the gate, we were given a parking spot on the grounds. We parked and went into Town Hall. We were given the VIP treatment, something we didn't expect. When we went in, we met with her staff and other council members. We were taken on a tour of the hall, and it was awe-inspiring. We were proud to be walking in a place with so much history, where some of our forefathers passed legislation for the rights and the values we have today. I'm sure they are rolling over in their graves for the way things turned out for Manny.

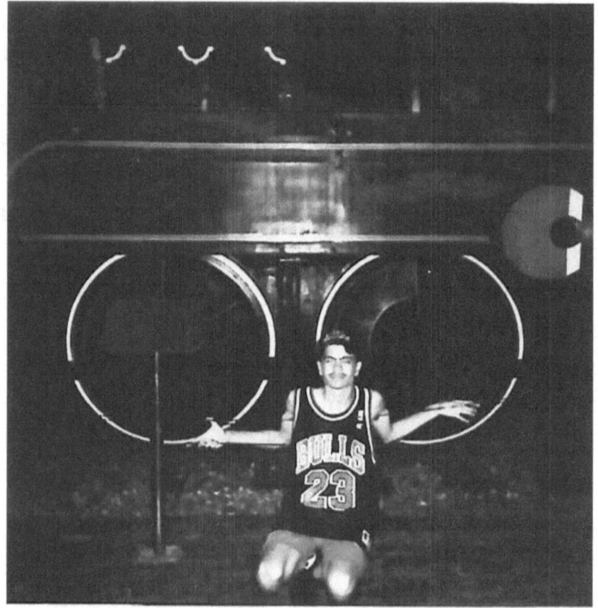

Manny in Back to the Future in Florida

After the tour was over, she came to meet us and first expressed her condolences. Then she vowed to pass a city law to prevent this from happening again. She asked us if we were aware that there were funds available to pay for Manny's care. We told her that we didn't. She wanted to know if anyone had told us about these funds. Again we said that they did not. She seemed to get angry about this fact. Then she vowed to us that she would put an end to this practice.

Then we went to a press conference where we were again introduced to the press. Ms. Quinn expressed her outrage and vowed to pass a law to prevent it from happening to anyone again. This was the first act that she did as the city council speaker. After the speeches were made, we again were interviewed by the press. After the interviews, we thanked Christine Quinn for her efforts. She thanked us for telling our story and making it public. Evidently, the city council has been trying to pass a law to prevent this type of horrors from happening, and because of us, now they would be able to make a push to make it so. The problem was that no one would make their story public. The average person is so distraught that they go into a shell and suffer silently. This is why the hospitals and doctors do this. No one would tell the world what they are doing, so for them it is business as usual. Well, they messed with the wrong family. We took our anguish and anger, and we channeled all those emotions to make sure that this would not be done to anyone again. We said our good-byes and thanked everyone involved, and we left.

So by this point we had an attorney, and we had the city council that wanted to pass a law in Manny's name. Manny's story had gone public. We were kind of numb by this point. We had to live through Manny' horror story over and over. It was quite an emotional ride, and this was just the beginning. This was taking its toll on Levia, who was now suffering asthma as a result of this. We were still in for an emotional roller coaster. Then we started suspecting that our phone was tapped. We started hearing clicking noises in the background, and we were hearing echoes of our voices every time we used the phone. How can we prove it? We kept asking ourselves over and over. Then we were told, "If you want to see if your phone is tapped, stop paying your bill." That was exactly what we did, and for an entire year, we didn't pay our bill. Guess what . . . our phone service was never terminated. We didn't even get a termination notice when the bills came every month. I kept putting the money aside if and when we finally did get a notice. But that didn't come until a year had passed.

I know what you're thinking. This guy is nuts; he's getting paranoid. Maybe so, but think about this. We were dealing with important elected officials on the state and federal level. We were dealing with the state health department. We were going against the doctors and hospitals that have powerful organizations behind them. We were rocking the boat, going against the status quo. They wanted to keep things the way they were. Who are we to bring attention to a serious situation that we face in this country, a broken-for-profit health-care system? Also, when can anyone not pay their phone bill for an entire year and not even get a termination notice? No one. That's who, but we did. Then when we did get the termination notice and we paid our bill, miraculously, the clicking and echoes stopped. Still think I'm nuts? So maybe this isn't compelling proof for you, but like I said, we suspected our phone was tapped. You be the judge and draw your own conclusions.

We met with our attorney Mitch Carlinsky, and we started our retainer. He was now officially our attorney. I was told that since I never officially adopted Manny, I could not be on the lawsuit, so only Levia could officially sue them. I was told in not so many words that I was a nobody. Of course, he never said that, but I sure felt it. This, as you can imagine, broke my heart. Now in hindsight this was a blessing in disguise. This is why I am able to tell the story. I could not be gagged. Anyway, Levia first had to become executrix of Manny' estate. So she signed what seemed to be an endless amount of paperwork to get the ball rolling. I at that time felt like the odd man out. But I get the last laugh. God was again at work in his way that at that time didn't make sense but now is crystal clear. So started the legal process that would last seven years. I will get to that a little later.

The Christmas holidays were upon us again. This was the first Christmas since Manny's passing. It was a very painful time for our entire family. We normally decorated the house with lights and decorations on the outside. That year, however, we didn't put up Christmas lights. In fact, we haven't done it since. We also normally decorated a ten-foot tree inside our living room. That year we weren't going to put up a tree, but we decided against it. We still had our younger son, now fifteen, who was alive, and it wasn't fair to him not to put up a tree. Not only that, Christmas was one of Manny's favorite holidays. He wouldn't want us to wallow in misery, and he would want us to live on. So we put up a smaller four-foot tree and tried to celebrate as best as we could. That particular Christmas was a blue Christmas; the life of our house was gone. New Year's Eve was also sad. After all, 2005 was a bad year, but we looked toward the New Year with anticipation.

Then January 6 came upon us, and it marked the one-year anniversary of Manny's passing. We got flowers and went to his grave. It was a bad day for us, and we were upset because we didn't have a headstone for him yet. One year later and all he had was a marker with his name and the dates that marked his birth and his death. The fact that he had died was depressing enough, but that he still didn't have a headstone just added insult to injury. We tried to get him a headstone, but they are quite expensive. We had buried him in a double grave. This was done because we didn't want anyone next to him. This required that we put a double headstone, not just a single one. This requirement was the cemetery's rules, not ours. So needless to say, we spent our time at the grave, praying and crying. It was a very melancholic day, to say the least.

We had a garage sale to try to raise money for Manny's headstone. We gathered personal items and received many donations from neighbors many that were left on our front porch. We raised nine hundred dollars at that sale but it was short of the tree thousand dollars we needed for the headstone. Then a neighbor that lives around the corner offered to have a fund raiser on our behalf. This lady was an acquaintance and we agreed.

It was to be held at a local bar that was off a major road by our house. The bar agreed to close for the day and not sell any liquor. This lady had had fund raisers there before and we reluctantly agreed with the location. There was to be a garage sale and I was to buy food to be sold at the event. I bought hot dogs and hamburgers and soft drinks.

We again received many donations from neighbors including fine artwork, clothing household items etc. We received donated chips from the local 7 eleven. Our local Dunkin Doughnuts donated doughnuts and coffee. Local businesses and antique shops donated knick knacks and fine antiques. We gathered an abundance of items.

We were told to drop off the items and food at the bar the morning of the event. We did as instructed and so it began. I was busy barbecuing the food and my wife was busy telling Manny's tragic story over and over. The event was huge people from all over attended. There was a live band and raffles of several donated items.

I sold all the food and drinks. And most of the garage sale items were sold. The raffle tickets were sold at a dollar a chance. All the tickets were put in bucket and all the items were raffled off. We didn't realize at the time but all the good items were won by friends of the lady running the event for us. Levia and I made the mistake of allowing the lady and her cronies to be in charge of the money, big mistake on our part.

At the end Levia was told to leave the items that were left over that they would tend to them. Levia sensed something was off and refused the offer. "I will pack it up and take it home" she said. At the end the lady handed Levia two hundred sixty six dollars and said that was all that was raised. Levia was furious she said "with all the food and items that was sold this is all there is?" To my wife's credit she held back her anger took the money and said nothing more.

She got into our car and I headed home. Then she said "honey we only raised two hundred sixty six dollars we got screwed!" I was furious I spent more than that on the food I bought. When we arrived home I parked the car in the garage and went inside. Levia however stayed in the garage a long time.

I stayed inside the house I was furious. I didn't want to fight with Levia after all it wasn't her fault. So I waited until I calmed down before I went to see what was keeping her. A short time later I went to the garage and she was hysterically crying. "They stole my baby's money!" she said. "They stole money from the dead!" she wailed. "I know they did" I replied. Then I went to her held her and we cried together.

We did finally get a headstone for his grave. It was given to us by Levia's childhood friend. She had given it to Levia as a birthday present. We shopped around and chose a place called Alan E. Fricke Memorials, and they made a beautiful headstone for our son. We picked an impala black granite stone. It has two roses on the upper right and left corner with a scroll that connected them. It has a cross in the top center. Where the family name is usually put, we decided to have written "May the force be with you" inside a beautiful ribbon with rose leaves surrounding the ribbon. There is another rose on the top-right section of the ribbon. Then on bottom left is written

"Manny" on the top line. The next line is MANUEL N. LANZA JR., and below that is JULY 9, 1980–JAN. 6, 2005. On the following line is *Beloved Son, Brother and Friend*, and under that on the space left over was placed as a gift from the memorial owner. They engraved *Star Wars Revenge of the Sith* exactly as it appears on the front cover of the DVD. The *III* is in gold leaf.

We were in constant contact with Christine Quinn, and she was keeping us up to date with the status of the law. She told us that the law was now going to be a state law. Thomas Duane, a New York senator, took the law up to Albany. We, as you can imagine, were thrilled about these turn of events. Manny's Law was going to be a New York State law. We spoke for a while, then we asked her what was taking so long for the health department to conduct their investigation. Christine told us she would look into the status for us. She wrote a letter to the health commissioner on our behalf.

The letter was dated January 11, 2006, and it read as follows:

Antonia C. Novello, M.D., M.P.H, Dr. P.H.,
Commissioner
New York State Department of Health
Corning Tower, Empire State Plaza
Albany, NY 12237

Dear Commissioner Novello:

Since the tragic death of Manuel Lanza, I have been in contact with his family. On their behalf I want to inquire about the two pending New York State Department of Health (NYDDOH) investigation regarding Manuel's death—one investigation involving St. Luke's-Roosevelt Hospital Center and the other involving Manuel Lanza's doctor at St. Luke's-Roosevelt Hospital Center.
I would appreciate it if you could inform Ms. Levia Prieto (Manuel's Mother) and me about where in the process NYSDOH is in the investi-

gations and what is the timeline for the completion of the investigations.

Below you will find the case numbers for the two investigations regarding the death of Manuel Lanza.

St. Luke's-Roosevelt Investigation - NY 00015909

Physician Investigation - OPMC NY-05-02-0799

Thank you for your assistance in this matter. If you have any questions, please feel to contact me Jeremy Hoffman at *his number here.*

Sincerely,
Christine C. Quinn
Speaker
New York City Council


cc: Levia Prieto

Then on February 3, 2006, we got an envelope delivered to our door. It was from the department of health. I signed for it, and I yelled out, "Honey, we got an envelope from the Department of Health!" I handed the envelope over to Levia, and she immediately opened it. We read the cover letter, which stated that they had found St. Luke's Roosevelt Hospital to be in violation of the New York State Hospital Code. They had issued a Statement of Deficiencies to the hospital enumerating its numerous and specific violations. In addition, the department is levying the maximum fine allowable under the law. Then we looked at the attached copy of Statement of Deficiencies. They had slapped the hospital with nine violations. Six were pertaining to Manny; the other three were not.

The six violations that pertained to Manny were as follows:

1. Failed to properly evaluate Lanza's severe brain ailment.
2. Allowed doctors to treat Lanza who misrepresented themselves as neurosurgeons when they were radiologists.

3. Never saw that Lanza was examined by a neurosurgeon, a specialist who could best evaluate his condition and recommend treatment.
4. Sent him home without adequate medication or a follow-up plan to monitor his life threatening condition.
5. Failed to keep complete records in Lanza's case, making it difficult to document and follow his treatment.
6. Discharged Lanza without evidence that a doctor evaluated him or discussed his severe condition with him and his family.

The other three violations were pertaining to other patients and had nothing to do with Manny. But because we brought Manny's inadequate care to light, they were found. So Manny was already saving lives of other people. The investigation did not find them in violation of federal dumping laws that required them to give emergency care. This law is known as EMTALA (Emergency Treatment and Labor Act); it was passed in 1986. This was very unfortunate.

The hospital was also slapped with $18,000 in fines. The law only allowed $2,000 per violation. That is appalling; this is a slap on the wrist. No wonder these types of things are happening. A $2,000 fine for an organization that deals in billions of dollars is a joke. That is like us getting fined a penny for a violation we may have committed. What is to prevent them from doing this again? Nothing, so again it's business as usual for these types of practices that occur much too often. The laws need to change; a much stiffer penalty must be put in place. I say more like at least a million dollars per offense. This might make them think twice. In addition, they should lose their accreditation for running a hospital. That would definitely make them think twice.

Well, this was a copy that was sent to us. The official announcement was not made yet. Levia and I figured that the public should be made aware of this immediately. So we called Sue Edelman at the *Post* and told her we got the report. We told her that the hospital was slapped with nine violations. She wanted us to send her a copy, which we did. She wanted to do a follow-up story for the Sunday edition of the *Post*. We sent her a copy immediately, and we waited for the Sunday edition.

Then on Sunday, February 5, 2006, we bought the *Post* early in the morning. There it was on page 2, the announcement to the world. The headlines read, "Hosp $lapped for tragic Manny Botch," with the story about the violations and the fines they had to pay. This was all done before the official announcement. The Department of Health wasn't pleased with our release, but to tell you the truth, I couldn't care less. After all, last June they dismissed the case, saying that he would have died anyway. This was a complete 180 from their initial ruling. See how persistence pays; the squeaky wheel gets the grease. Take it from me. Don't let the system dictate things. If an injustice has occurred, keep putting the pressure on until the truth comes out. The truth is the truth, and nothing can prevent it from coming to light. Like one of my son's favorite song says, pursue the truth no matter where it lies. That lyric kept playing over and over in our minds like a loop through this whole ordeal.

This I know annoyed Dr. Novello. She wanted to have her own official announcement. We took the winds out of her sails. Quite honestly, I couldn't care less about how she felt. After all, she wasn't the one who lost a loved one. Besides, if the story had not gone public, then Manny's case would have been swept under the rug and forgotten. I can only wonder how many unfortunate families this was done to. She wanted this situation to go away, but we weren't going to allow it. Too bad for her!

Then on February 7, 2006, another article was printed in the *Post*. The headlines read, "Commish's Manny Rx for state hosps," again written by Sue Edelman. This article was where Dr. Novello was vowing to push for reforms that would guarantee that no other New Yorker is denied proper hospital treatment over lack of insurance. She was urging for laws that would require hospitals to inform the uninsured that charity care is available, to help uninsured patients apply for Medicaid or financial aid. She wanted hospitals to pay stiffer fines, more than the current $2,000 per violation, when patients died because of shoddy care. Then she expressed sympathy to our family and said how she was brokenhearted. This was her way of saving face; she is a phony.

There was also a statement made by the hospital, which they stated that they were glad they weren't found to have violated federal dumping laws. "In fact," they said, "care was provided to Mr. Lanza by St. Luke's Roosevelt despite his lack of insurance. St. Luke's Roosevelt and its medical staff met the highest standards of medical ethics."

Really? They did nothing for him while he was there! The hospital also noted that Manny was evaluated by a neurosurgeon at Brookhaven Hospital on Long Island before being transferred to Roosevelt. Manny was seen by a neurosurgeon at Brookhaven, but they are located more than sixty miles away. The key word in that statement is transferred. St. Luke's Roosevelt took charge of Manny's care when they accepted him as a patient. They should have had one of their neurosurgeons evaluate Manny, but they didn't. If they, as they claimed, met the highest standard of medical ethics, then I would hate to know what they considered the lowest standard was. This is a frightening thought.

Like I said before, I worked at a hospital as a pharmacy technician. I am well aware that if, for example, you are a cardiac patient who has had a heart attack and seen by a cardiologist, if that facility is not able to give the proper care and if they transfer him/her to another facility, then the other facility takes charge for the care of that person. They are reevaluated by the new facility's cardiologist. What I am saying is, the new cardiologist now takes charge of the patient. The only time this is not done is when the original cardiologist has privileges to treat at the new facility. Manny's neurosurgeon did not have privileges to treat at St. Luke's Roosevelt. So their statement was false, and it was said because most people are not aware of this fact. Manny should have been reevaluated by a neurosurgeon at St. Luke's.

On April 26, 2006, the Patient Information Act, known as Manny's Law, was signed into law. Governor Pataki, who was the governor at that time, signed the bill under the table. He didn't want any more bad press for this debacle. So we were not able as a family to have another press conference and be present for the signing. This is usually done when a law is signed in honor of the person that the law was named after. This was a little disheartening for us. But since we gave the state a black eye, I guess this was our punishment.

We felt that Manny should have been honored. After all, he was the one that died simply because he had gotten sick. It wasn't his fault that no one wanted to care for him. The fact that the Department of Health tried to dismiss his case initially was not his fault, or ours for that matter. The fact that an incompetent commissioner was in charge of the health department was Pataki's fault, not ours. We were getting conflicting reports that the law was known as the Patient Information Act and not Manny's Law, so we asked our attorney, Mitch Carlinsky, to write Governor Pataki on our behalf, which he did. He sent the letter, and as expected, we got no response to the letter.

Then we asked Christine Quinn for a copy of the law. She graciously sent us a very fancy copy of the law. It was on thick yellow-tinged (like antique) paper with the New York State seal on the top. The Assembly and Senate of the State of New York was printed below the state seal. Under that was "Manny's Law," and under that was S. 6457-C, A. 9557-B, which represented the bill numbers in the appropriate chamber in Albany. Now we see for sure that it is named Manny's Law. Then there were seven pages of the law in detail. The law was to take effect January 1, 2007. The highlights of the law are as follows:

1) The law requires hospitals to inform uninsured patients or patients that have exhausted their health insurance of charity care and financial aid available to them. To post this information in conspicuous places of congregation.

2) That the hospital could no longer charge more than what highest volume payer pays for such services. (This means that they cannot charge more that the amount paid by the insurance that paid them the most claims the previous calendar year.)

3) Patients with income levels below the 100% poverty level will be charged a nominal fee (a fraction of normal amount) as consistent with commissioner guidelines.

4.  Patient with income of 100–150% of federal poverty level can be charged on a sliding scale where lower income pays lowest amount (nominal fee) up to no more than 20% of highest volume payer (example, if the highest amount paid is $1,000, you cannot be charged more than $200 for said service).

5)  Patients with incomes from 151–250% of poverty level where the lowest pays less on a sliding scale from 20% up to 100% of amount paid by highest volume payer.

6)  Patients with incomes from 251–300% can be charged no more than what the highest volume payer normally pays for said service.

7)  Repayment plans cannot exceed 10% of gross income.

8)  Primary residence, tax deferred or comparable retirement accounts, college savings account, or cars used regularly can no longer be considered assets and used against patients.

As a direct result of Manny's Law, some examples of the flat fee for individuals at or below the federal poverty level and who meet certain asset requirements are guaranteed specific low costs for certain services, as set by the NYSDOH. Hospitals cannot charge qualifying patients more than $150 for ambulatory surgery. They cannot charge more than $150 for MRI testing or more than $15 for adult emergency room/clinic services. If this law was in effect when Manny was alive, he would have been able to get a discounted price for his services, instead of the $42,000 dollars that he was billed for the inadequate care that he received.

This amount, by the way, was being charged by the parties involved after his death, even when they were told he had died. They came after us to pay up. Technically, we weren't responsible for payment. Manny was an adult under the law, and he was considered an independent, but that didn't stop them. Brookhaven Hospital went as far as to use a collection agency called POM to put a lien on Manny's estate. Can you imagine? When we told our attorney about the lien, he simply stated, "Let them try." When the story went public, one by one they stopped collection because of all the bad press they were getting. Even Brookhaven finally stopped, but they were the last. This is a common practice for hospitals when they really don't need to do this. They can get reimbursed from the funds available from the state. Shame on them!

I don't think it is fair that if a person is paying for care in cash, they should pay so much more than a person who has insurance. If insurance is paying, say, one hundred dollars to a doctor, then why should you as a cash patient pay five hundred dollars for the same care? Why should you pay a hospital two thousand dollars a day for each day in the hospital in cash, when the insurance pays the seven hundred and fifty dollars for the same care? That doesn't sound fair, and there should be laws that prevent this, and we as a nation should stand up and stop this unfair practice. An example is if you go to a gas station to fill up your car, you usually pay ten cents less per gallon for cash, not more because you are a cash-paying customer, which is what our health-care system does. If a doctor agrees to be paid one hundred dollars by an insurance company, then he should not charge more than a hundred dollars for cash. Think about it.

The law of course is only for New York State residents in New York hospitals that have emergency rooms. The law isn't perfect, but it's a step in the right direction. Levia and I have informed many people of the law. My wife always had copies of the law in her purse. We gave them to people who were having issues with their health care. We have even been thanked for the information because it led to a patient previously being denied care now getting the care they needed. So we know that Manny has saved several lives. Of course the law does not include doctors in private practice. We have held forums in our local library and our local civic association. We have been interviewed by our local town papers all in the effort to inform the public that Manny's Law exist. Although we tirelessly try to inform the public about the law, we are just three people. Manny's Law should be posted beside the patient bill of rights. Now we put our hopes that universal health care in this country becomes a reality.

Well, the law has become a reality, thanks to the efforts of Christine Quinn, Speaker of the NYC Council, and State Senator Thomas Duane and State Assembly Member Pete Grannis. We would like to thank them from the bottom of our hearts. You guys have made a difficult time a little more bearable. You saw the pain and anguish in our hearts, and you showed us compassion. You made sure Manny did not die in vain. You guys will never be forgotten either by me or my family ever. You hold a special place in our hearts.

About six months later, Christine Quinn decided to check up on the hospitals. She wanted to see if they were doing what was required by the law. So she had her staff start visiting and calling hospitals to see if they were in fact telling people that charity care or financial aid was available. So they conducted an investigation and started checking on the city hospitals. After the investigation was completed and all the findings were tabulated, we again were asked to attend another press conference at city hall.

So on October 30, 2007, we went to the city hall. We arrived at 10:30 a.m. as was asked, and again we were treated like VIPs. This again was an honor. We met with the staff and Christine Quinn, and we went over the results of the investigations before it was made public, and she gave us a copy. Then we went out to the conference room and to yet another press conference. Speeches were made by Levia and me; we thanked Christine Quinn and expressed the importance of Manny's Law. Then Ms. Quinn announced the checkup that was made and then told everyone the results of the report. We again were all over the airwaves and the papers. The following is a copy of the highlights of the report that we received:

## Executive Summary

The number of uninsured Americans has hit its highest level since 1999, with 2.2 million more Americans, including 600,000 more children, identifying as uninsured. According to the New York City Department of Health and Mental Hygiene (DOHMH), one million adult New Yorkers, about 1 in 6, do not have health insurance. In 2005, uninsured Long Island resident Manny Lanza died because he didn't receive needed treatment from a New York hospital reportedly due to his inability to pay. This report analyzes the effectiveness of "Manny's Law," a new State law, designed to help the most vulnerable of uninsured New Yorkers. Manny's Law requires all New York State hospitals to develop and administer a financial assistance program as a condition of receiving funding from the $847 million New York State Bad Debt and Charity Care, and Disproportional Share pool. The law went into effect in January 2007, and hospitals received guidance from the New York State Department of Health in late June 2007. While this investigation finds that most New York City hospitals provide patients information about their financial assistance programs when asked, it also shows a need for increased hospital staff training, and stricter enforcement and regulations on how hospital should follow certain aspects of the law.

This report will:

(1)  Demonstrate that most hospitals in New York City offer information to prospective patients about their financial assistance programs;
(2)  Illustrate inconsistencies in how hospitals determine where to post signs about their financial assistance programs and provide information regarding these programs;
(3)  Highlights the need for the New York State Department of Health to issue regulations for how hospitals should execute certain aspects of the law.

## Key Findings

### Signage

Manny's Law requires hospitals with 24-hour emergency departments to notify patients of their financial assistance programs through "conspicuous posting of language-appropriate information in the general hospital." Investigators surveyed ten common and conspicuous areas of each hospital and noted whether posters about financial assistance were displayed.

Of the 59 hospitals visited:

(1)  13 hospitals (22%) had no signs posted.
(2)  9 hospitals (15%) had posters in only 1 area.

(3)   1 hospital (2%) had posters in all areas surveyed.

(4)   37 hospitals (63%) had posters in 2 or more areas surveyed.

Verbal information about Manny's Law

In site visits and phone calls, investigators surveyed billing office staff in an effort to simulate the experience an uninsured patient might encounter inquiring about how to pay for care.

(1)   Staff at 42 hospitals (74%) told investigators about financial assistance without Prompting;

(2)   Staff at 5 hospitals (9%) told investigators about financial assistance program only when prompted;

(3)   Staff at 9 hospitals (16%) never told investigators about their financial assistance program, even after prompting, including staff at 5 hospitals (9%) who said that a patient could not receive care if he/she were not able to pay.

## Phone Surveys

During the 58 hospital billing office phone surveys:

(1)   Staff at 43 hospitals (74%) told investigators about their financial assistance program without prompting;

(2)   Staff at 8 hospitals (14%) told investigators about their financial assistance program when prompted;

(3)   Staff at 4 hospitals (7%) never told investigators about their financial assistance program, even after prompting, including 2 hospitals (3%), who said that a patient could not receive care if he/she were unable to pay.

## Recommendations

It appears that most New York City hospitals are complying with Manny's Law provisions about signage and patient notification. However, there still remain potential barriers to accessing these programs, either because of the inconsistency of staff training or because a lack of definition in the State law. The City Council's recommendations therefore focus on ways that hospitals can increase knowledge of and access to these programs.

(1) The New York State Department of Health (DOH) should conduct annual random checks of hospitals to evaluate compliance with the State law and accessibility of their financial assistance program.

DOH needs to continue oversight of hospital financial assistance programs by proactively ensuring that hospitals have not only created a financial assistance policy, but also are complying with State law by hanging posters and providing information to consumers.

(2) The New York Department of Health should develop regulations that define the "conspicuous places" that poster must be placed.

DOH has made recommendations to hospitals about the locations to place financial assistance posters, but DOH should develop stricter and enforceable regulations that require hospitals in specific conspicuous areas, like the ER and clinic waiting rooms.

(3) All New York hospitals should conduct further staff training on their financial assistance programs.

Staff responses to investigators' phone calls and site visits show a need for hospitals to train billing office staff, as well as other hospital staff to ensure that all individuals interacting with patients are aware of the hospital's financial assistance program and how patients can apply.

(4) Hospitals should follow the State Department of Health sample assistance application. All hospitals should evaluate their applications to make sure they are asking only for necessary information.

This investigation was done, and it only pertained to New York City hospitals. That was Christine Quinn's jurisdiction. This doesn't include New York State hospitals. God only knows how the report would have read if they were included. Can you imagine that several hospitals still said that if a patient cannot afford to pay, he couldn't be treated? Now the report graciously stated that maybe it was because of improper training of staff. No . . . This was the normal thing that was done, and these hospitals were doing business as usual. No money or insurance, too bad, no treatment. If it costs an individual his/her life, sucks for you. Of course now it has been difficult to keep track of the status of the law. Christine Quinn is no longer the Speaker. She did try to become mayor of New York City, but unfortunately, she lost the election. Levia did the commercial for Ms. Quinn, who was considered the front runner for the mayor's position at that time.

I personally used to push for her becoming mayor. My work brings me into the city often, and I would tell everyone I came into contact with to vote for her. Unfortunately, the people voted for De Blasio, who was an underqualified individual that had no prior experience in public office. He was a public advocate, and that does not qualify a person for running a city as large as the Big Apple. I can tell you from experience that the Big Apple is in disarray. The traffic jams are horrendous because of all the construction that he is doing simultaneously all over the city and at the height of rush hour. The police department does not respect him; in fact, they hate him. His approval rating as of June 2016 is 35 percent. Now he has election finance problems. Allegedly some funny business went on when he ran for mayor. Allegedly some of his campaign contributions have been questioned about their legality. In my opinion, Christine Quinn would have been a far superior choice, but that is just my opinion. Sorry, Christine, I hope all is well with you.

Now we come to the lawsuit. Let me tell you, that was a long and grueling process that took seven years to come to a conclusion. I first want to say to the attorneys that represented the doctors and hospital, shame on you. How can you in good conscience be of counsel to greedy doctors that broke their oath as doctors and a greedy hospital who neglected my son? You guys, in my opinion, are the scum of the earth that would sell their souls for money. To the doctors, shame on you for breaking your oath. Who are you to play God and decide who lives and who dies?

First, Levia had to be made the executrix or representative of Manny's estate, as I stated earlier. Then our attorney had to find a neurologist or neurosurgeon to agree that Manny's care was not up to medical standards. This was easier said than done. Mitch had a tough time trying to find one. We needed a doctor in order to file a lawsuit. It seemed that no doctor was willing to go against them. Neurology is a small field, and I guess they all know each other, and no one up to this point was willing to step up to plate. Finally, Mitch found a neurologist that was retiring and was willing to not only sign an affidavit but also to testify if needed against them. Then on Friday, June 2, 2006, Mitch filed a wrongful-death lawsuit against St. Luke's Roosevelt Hospital and three doctors.

Let me tell you about New York State wrongful death law. New York requires proof of five elements:

(1) Death
(2) Caused by the wrongful conduct of the defendant
(3) Proving a cause of action the deceased may have pursued in court if the death had not occurred
(4) Survived by one or more persons who have suffered a loss as the result of the death
(5) Damages the estate can recover

The responsibility for filing a wrongful death claim falls on the shoulders of the personal representative that is approved by the court of the deceased person's estate. This person then disperses the award to any heir or beneficiaries to whomever he/she sees fit. Damages that can be claimed are as follows:

(1) Funeral and burial expenses
(2) Reasonable medical, nursing, and other health-care expenses related to the person that died, person's final injury or illness
(3) Wages and benefits lost between the deceased person's final injury or illness and his or her death
(4) Lost inheritance suffered by surviving children

> (5)  Pain and suffering endured by the deceased due to the
> final injury or illness

And wrongful death claim must be filed within two years of the date of the deceased person's death. The survivors cannot claim pain and suffering for themselves for his loss.

In our case, since Manny wasn't married and didn't have children and since the mother and brother were the only survivors (remember, I didn't count), the amount that could be awarded was limited because it was dependent on the amount Manny could've contributed to us while he was alive. Meaning since he was twenty-four years old, it was assumed that he would eventually marry and leave our household. So how much can Manny have contributed to us? Also, since Manny died so soon after the onset of his diagnosis, how much could he have suffered? Basically, he was worth more if he would have been married or if he would have had children. We were bringing this lawsuit not for the money; Manny was priceless. We were doing this because the only way they would feel our pain was if we reached into their pockets and took money from them. They were about the money.

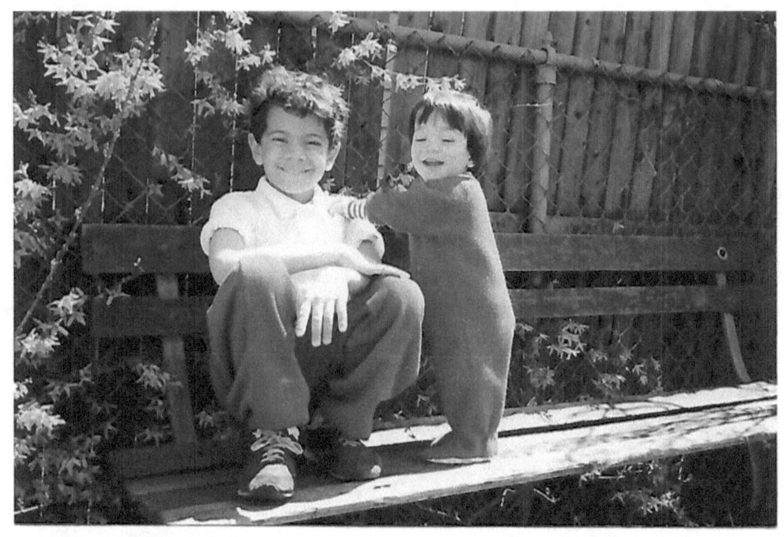

Manny's Favorite cousin James Scozzari young

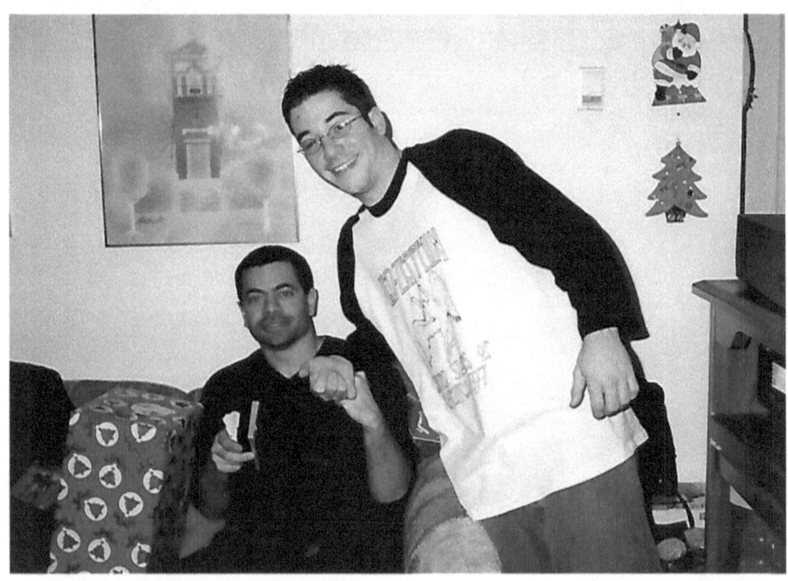

James Scozzari ESQ and his favorite cousin Manny older

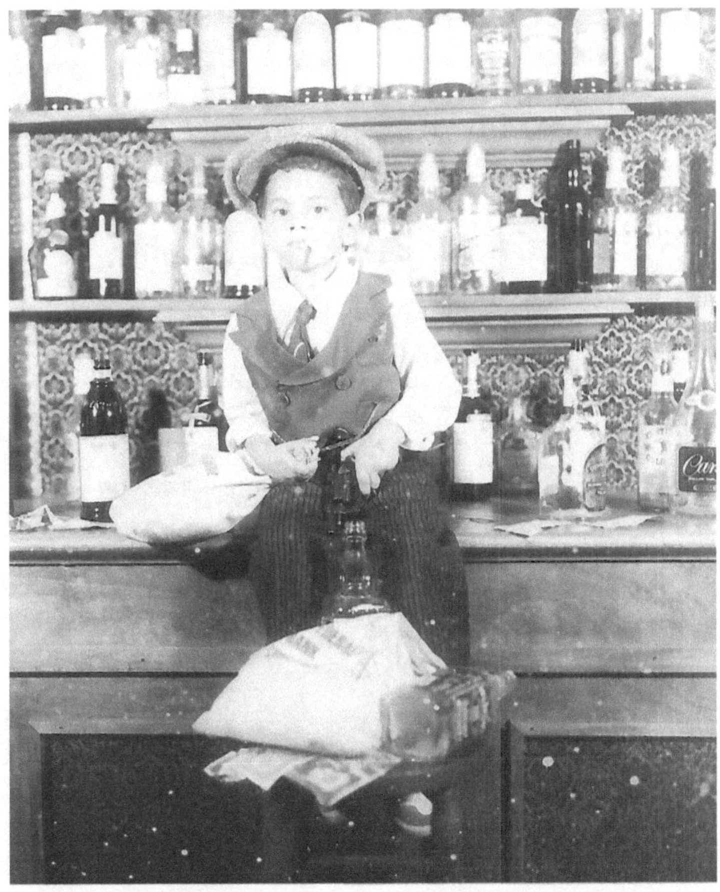

Manny at Wildwood New Jersey. This is an old fashion picture popular at the park he was very angry that they put the cigarette in his mouth

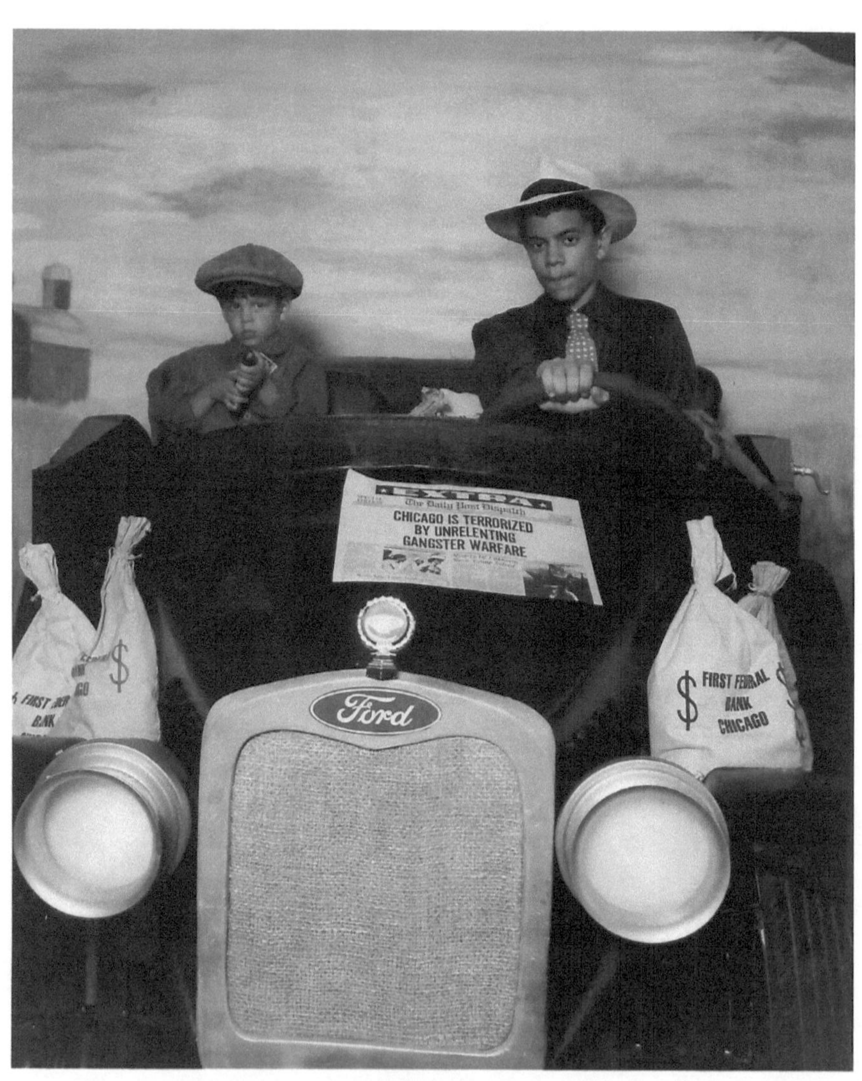


Manny and Kenneth as Wildwood New Jersey Time cut short

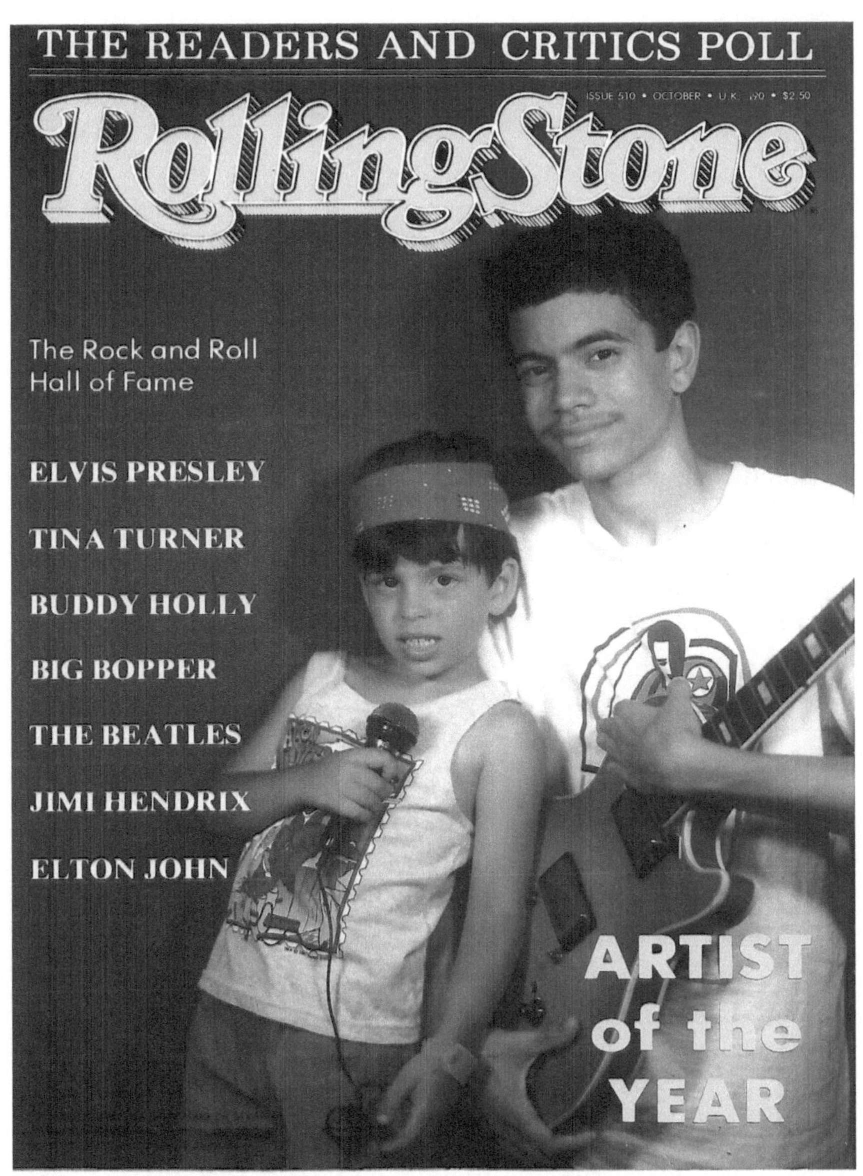


Manny and Kenneth at Wildwood isn't this one great

Now we entered what is the "discovery" stage of the lawsuit. This is the stage where the attorneys from both sides prepare their case. The evidence was presented by our side and given to their side. This is done so that they can prepare a defense for their client. Then all the medical records are scrutinized. The autopsy is also scrutinized. Depositions or statements are taken from the parties involved. Basically, both sides are preparing for trial by jury. Sounds easy, but it's time-consuming, and it took about two years to go to this stage. I can't tell you how many times their story changed. Our story, however, never changed; it stayed just as you read it. The truth is the truth, and it never changes. They kept grasping at straws, trying to justify that there was no error in what they had done. Every time they opened their mouths, they inserted their foot into it, looking like the imbeciles that they are. They kept changing their reasoning over and over, and each time they sounded sillier with each change of their story.

The first thing their attorney tried to do was to try to get our evidence thrown out and become inadmissible. With every motion they filed with the courts, trying to get evidence thrown out, each and every time the judge would deny their motion. It was ruled that all the evidence that our attorney presented to the court was allowed to be presented in court. This I'm sure was frustrating to their attorneys. These attorneys were fools for trying to clear the doctors and hospital of any wrongdoing. Like I said before, shame on them for representing the doctors and hospital.

The defendants' (their) attorney filed a motion to have the case dismissed. They were of the contention that there was no casual connection for this AVM and Manny's death. They believed that the element of causation (or cause) is missing and the plaintiff (our attorney) would be unable to prove causation at a trail. They urged the court to dismiss the case because of the failure to make this connection. The motion also cited that Dr. Berenstein (one of the defendants) in a sworn affidavit said that Manny did not die from his AVM. His opinion was that since he didn't hemorrhage and since this was the most common reason a person dies from an AVM, it didn't cause his death. He also stated that seizures can also cause death, but that it was rare. And since there was no evidence of this in the autopsy, a seizure also did not cause his death. Basically, because of this, he said the medical examiner was wrong in her autopsy report.

Our attorney argued that if Manny had been treated in a timely fashion, then his risk factors would have been reduced so that, more probable than not, he would have not died from his AVM. We supported our argument with affirmation from a neurologist who supported our side. He reviewed all medical records, the autopsy reports, as well as the defendant's depositions and the affidavit from Dr. Berenstein.

He first points out that the autopsy report itself indicates AVM as the cause of death. He further pointed out that Dr. Berenstein himself acknowledged that a seizure could cause death. He then described a syndrome known as SUDEP, which stands for sudden unexpected death in epilepsy. He went on to state that a number of patients who die from this syndrome have no abnormal findings in an autopsy. He further stated that the autopsy report did indicate a frothy material was found in Manny's lungs. He added that it is well-known that patients that have epileptic seizures have frothy secretions in their oral cavities and lungs.

So it was his opinion with a reasonable degree of medical certainty that Manny suffered a seizure and that was what caused his death. And with regard to the frothy material found in the lungs, that Dr. Berenstein was wrong when he stated that there was no evidence of seizure or secondary effects of seizure, because there were. He then discussed the plan that the doctors and the hospital had recommended for Manny, which consisted of palliative treatments involving staged embolization so as to shrink the AVM and then treat it with radiosurgery. It was his medical opinion that the delay in commencing treatments, or any other treatments for that matter, was a deviation from accepted medical care. Finally he expressed his opinion that Manny's lack of insurance coverage played a part in the delays of these treatments.

In reply, the defense counsel took issue with the neurologist's opinion that a seizure caused by the AVM caused his death. Counsel argued that the doctor who performed the autopsy merely noted a small amount of red foam in the bronchi, which is different from frothy material in his lungs. Counsel argued that this is a material exaggeration. With regard to the issue of seizures, counsel made the argument that the defendants had nothing to do with the seizures that he first began experiencing in September 2004. Rather, it was Dr. Sabrina Johnson at the health center who was following and treating Manny for his condition. Therefore, the defendants should not be charged with malpractice if the seizure were the cause of death.

The judge found this last argument unconvincing. It is foolish to suggest that the defendants' overall plan to provide palliative treatment so as to drastically reduce the size of the AVM and to try to excise (remove) it would have nothing to do with the treatment of the seizure symptom of the AVM. Seizures here were very possibly related to the AVM, so a plan to deal with the AVM would of course be dealing with the symptoms from that AVM as well.

With regard to the exaggeration of the medical examiner's autopsy findings, the judge did not believe that such exaggeration led to the rejection of the neurologist's opinion that there was some evidence of a red foam caused from a fatal seizure. As he pointed out, some seizures show no evidence whatsoever in an autopsy. There was something small showing here.

Finally, one has to consider here that medical examiner who conducted the autopsy and wrote the report had the opinion that the cause of death here was cerebral arteriovenous malformation. The judge believed in her opinion, as expressed in an official autopsy report, and it must be given some consideration, particularly because the defendants express no opinion as to why or from what Mr. Lanza died.

In the last analysis, the judge was obliged to give the neurologist's opinion some weight, since he was a credentialed neurologist who had reviewed all the relevant records in the case and held the opinion as to the cause of death with a reasonable degree of medical certainty. His opinion was that a seizure caused by Manny's AVM caused his death. The neurologist did point out that the defendant doctors did connect AVM with seizures. It should also be noted that Mr. Lanza first appeared at Brookhaven Hospital due to seizures and loss of consciousness.

Therefore, the judge concluded that there was an issue of fact as to the causation (cause) between the AVM and the alleged delay of treatment for it and Mr. Lanza's death. So the defendants' motion for summary judgment (dismissal) was denied.

I would like to state that Dr. Johnson was not Manny's primary physician; they were. Also, she was not treating him for his condition; they were. She was monitoring his Dilantin levels, and she made sure he had enough medicine, which they didn't. Neurology was not her expertise; she was just a general practitioner. Besides, she was the only one that was willing to help us. For them to suggest that she was responsible was ludicrous. What a bunch of fools to even suggest this. They were just grasping at straws.

Then the day arrived that my wife had to give her deposition or statement that would be presented to the court. We drove into Queens to an attorney's office that Mitch was using as "of counsel" to our trial. We all gathered in the office and were introduced to Michael Binder, who was the attorney that was "of counsel" on our side. Then we went into the conference room. I was allowed to be present as long as I stayed quiet throughout the proceedings. I wasn't allowed to say anything or utter any sound or show signs of approval or disapproval to any statement made. Then the court reporter came in and sat by the stenotype machine. That is the machine that a court reporter uses to type what a person says and keeps an official record of it and is presented to the court. Then their attorney entered, and she came in with arrogance, like she was a goddess. She might have thought she was a goddess, but she had no idea that the Almighty God Jehovah was on our side.

She sat down, and we were introduced to her. I got to say, she seemed to be very full of herself. I wasn't impressed. The attorneys went through the rules and told Levia to wait for the question to be completely asked before giving an answer. She was told to speak slowly and clearly so the court reporter could hear and keep an accurate account of the statements made. Then they asked if she understood what was going to happen and what her statement were to be used for. Levia answered that she understood.

The deposition started; the attorneys gave their names for the record. Then the questions started, and Levia answered them slowly and clearly. Their attorney tried her best to trip Levia up, but she stood her ground and never wavered from the truth. Their side kept trying to make it look like it was Levia's fault that Manny died. Every time Levia gave an answer that their attorney didn't like, she would say, "Strike that," which she said quite often. This meant that that statement was to be stricken or omitted from the record. I thought that was a lot of bull, but this is the way things are done. I think this is a little unfair, but that's only my opinion. You be the judge. Levia gave her statement, as lopsided as it was. Then their attorney got up and left. She, in my opinion, seemed annoyed and she left. Good riddance. It was finally over, and I was proud of Levia. She stood firm in her resolve and told the truth, and she never lost her composure.

Then almost on a weekly basis, we had to keep hearing their lame excuses, which they changed constantly, as to why Manny died. First, they said that the medical examiner was wrong and Manny didn't die from his AVM. The judge asked them, if he didn't die from the AVM, then what did this young man die from? To this they could never give a definitive answer. Their story kept changing, but our story stayed the same.

Then they came up with the lame excuse that Manny had Hodgkin's disease. This is a type of cancer that affects the lymph nodes. In Manny's autopsy, it stated that his spleen had nodules (abnormal growth) consistent with sclerosing Hodgkin's disease. This means that he might or might not have developed Hodgkin's lymphoma. We will get to this in more detail later. They were using this as an excuse, but this was not what caused his death. The autopsy clearly stated that he died as a result of his AVM. So the judge didn't buy this excuse.

Then they used the excuse that Manny's AVM wasn't curable. This might be true, but it was in fact treatable. The fact that they didn't keep track of him, how could they know what condition he was in and if in fact he was getting worse? They just didn't care. They were just more concerned about getting paid than treating the patient. The judge didn't accept this excuse either. They just kept saying that his condition wasn't an emergency. Really? If this was true, then why did he die from his AVM? I'll tell you why. His condition was serious, and it should have been treated as an emergency.

Then on December 11, 2007, we received an envelope in the mail from Mitch's office. It was the result of the findings of our complaint of the doctors. There were many inconsistencies in this report. First, the report says at 1545 on 9/l 7, the ER nurse at Brookhaven wrote a note indicating that the patient would not be transferred then because "patient Medicaid pending" and that patient lost bed to another patient. What they omitted is that after Medicaid pending, it says, "And they have an issue with that." Then it says he lost bed to another patient. They conveniently omitted this.

Then on 9/18 the neurosurgeon wrote that the patient was neurologically stable, and there was no need for emergent neurosurgical intervention with drain. Then on 9/19 the medical attending wrote that the patient needed emergent medical care and was awaiting bed at St. Luke's. So which was it? He didn't need or he needed emergent (emergency) care? Remember that they were going to discharge him the next day. After I told the doctor that if anything happened to Manny I was going to hold him personally responsible, that was on 9/18/2004. Then the next day, 9/19 they made a 180 and stated that he did require emergent care. But of course, the doctors at St. Luke's said his care was not emergent. How would they know a neurosurgeon never evaluated him at St. Luke's? If it wasn't an emergency, then why did he die of his AVM? This report basically said that Manny wasn't denied care because of lack of insurance. This again shows that his complaint was shoved under the table. The hospital was slapped with violations, but the doctors were not, even though the report said that they misrepresented themselves. That in and of itself is a violation, is it not? This just shows the corruption and flaws in the system!

This is why we can't have doctors investigate doctors. The system just doesn't work. The doctors see themselves in a similar situation, and they don't find fault. Basically, what I am saying is that they cover each other's fault. This way, if they run into a similar situation, they too would be exonerated. This is a pretty convenient system for the doctors. Doctors can't investigate doctors. Just like police can't investigate police and politicians can't investigate politicians, etc. You see it all the time, like when police shoot an unarmed person and unjustly fire twenty-two shots at him. Then when they investigate, they are found not to be at fault. It is just a flawed system that needs to be changed.

We as citizens of the United States have got to put an end to all this corruption. We have to stand against injustice and demand change. We have the power to do this. Hey, we got a law passed, didn't we? We stood up against the establishment and prevailed. This was done by just two individuals. Imagine what we could do as a nation and we worked together to fix the system for the better. Then we would be a better people for it!

The doctors each gave their depositions, and of course, they kept saying that that Manny's condition wasn't an emergency. They insisted that they did everything by the book. Dr. Niimi did admit in his deposition that he did tell Mary that until Manny's Medicaid was in place, the procedure would not be scheduled. See, he admitted it; insurance was indeed an issue. But mostly their depositions were blah blah blah! Techno babble! These depositions were just a formality; at least Dr. Niimi admitted that he was waiting for Medicaid. They kept trying to show that they did nothing wrong. They kept insisting that Manny's case wasn't an emergency. Then again I ask them, "Really! Then why did he die?" A seizure is a sign that something is wrong. This was their way of trying to brush the blame elsewhere.

Name: Manuel Lanza
11/24/04
Call to patient

The patient has a diagnosis of a brain AVM and is to be scheduled for angiogram. Per Dr. Niimi, when the patient has his insurance in place (Medicaid), the procedure will be scheduled. This information was given to patient's mother who said that Medicaid is still not in place. She was given instructions to call Ms. Rose with the Medicaid information and numbers when they are available She will inform our staff when he maybe scheduled for admission.

Mary Madrid, RN, PhD

This was presented as evidence marked as exhibit 2 in the lawsuit. Dr. Niimi admitted under oath at the deposition that he did say this.

The above note was a crucial part of the evidence in our case. So of course their attorneys tried to get it thrown out and make it inadmissible in the trial. They filed a motion in limine. This is a motion asking the court for a ruling limiting or preventing certain evidence for being presented in court. They said that it was prejudicial to their client and should not be presented to the jury. I won't get into detail because the proceedings were long and I don't want to bore you. In summary, both sides presented their arguments. The judge weighed the evidence, and she decided that it was in fact part of the official medical records. Therefore, she denied the motion. This made it possible to present this evidence to the jury in trial.

If they were worried about this being prejudicial to their client, then maybe they shouldn't have made insurance an issue at all. We basically argued the point that after the angiogram was done on November 4, they initially scheduled him for November 11. This was one week after the angiogram, and then it was cancelled. Then they didn't schedule another appointment until February 5, 2005, three months later, because insurance was in some part an issue to the delay. Mitch stated that several calls were made to try to schedule it for an earlier date, and all that was mentioned was insurance, insurance, insurance. The judge acknowledged that both the hospital and doctors knew Manny didn't have insurance. She did believe that this was a factor, if even a small part, to the decision to wait for three months.

Then the issue of the Dilantin came up. Their side argued that this wasn't an insurance issue and that in fact they didn't have to give him the necessary care. Partly because we lived on Long Island and we were unable to make the appointments. Can you imagine how silly that sounds? We would have swum across the Atlantic Ocean and back to get Manny the care he needed. Besides, I own a car, and I am well able to get Manny to any appointment that was made. The judge cited that the DOH found violations concerning the Dilantin and also not providing the necessary follow-up care, that they went against the standard guidelines of standard of care. So she believed that insurance was in fact an issue concerning the delays. Anyway, basically their attorney every time he opened his month, inserted his foot in it. In the end, we could present our evidence, prejudicial or not.

Then they even tried to make it look like it was our fault. They were using the appointment that was made to meet with them and discuss his care. They stood by the position that we were the ones who cancelled the appointment, when it was them that actually cancelled it due to foul weather. Why in the world would we cancel an appointment that we so desperately tried to make? Levia and I would do anything possible to save Manny's life. Anyway, they were going to tell us risks of Manny's procedure at the appointment and justify their delays. They had no intentions of treating Manny sooner. We were the ones that were trying to get Manny cared for sooner. This was a position that they hung on to. Until the judge told them that wasn't a valid excuse. So their defense started crumbling, and little by little it collapsed, so much for their high-priced attorneys. Like I said before, I wasn't impressed with them in the first place.

The judge kept asking their attorneys what the reason was that this twenty-four-year-old young man died. Remember that they said that the medical examiner was wrong and that Manny didn't die of an AVM. No matter how many hearings they had, they never gave a definitive answer to that question. I know the answer to this. *They* were the reason Manny died. Then finally she gave up on them and told their attorney, "I think it's in your clients' best interest to come up with a monetary figure and settle this case." Imagine that the judge basically told them to pay up. Their manufactured and flawed defense had finally collapsed like a house of cards. So much for high-priced Manhattan-based lawyers.

Then in May of 2013, Mitch called Levia and told her that they had made an offer. The amount wasn't as much as you may imagine. Remember the wrongful death law? Our attorney negotiated a bit more, but again it was basically a slap on the wrist. The hospital insurance paid the claim. This way the doctors' malpractice insurance wouldn't go up in price. So it's business as usual for them. On October 15, 2013, Levia received her settlement check. The lawsuit took seven years to conclude and eight years after Manny's death. It was quite an emotional roller-coaster ride. At least they didn't get away with it. It wasn't about the money anyway.

It pains me that Manny was treated like he was an outcast, like his life was worthless. He wasn't worthless; he was priceless. He was a conscientious person that was always thinking of others. He would help others even if he had to make sacrifices to accomplish it. He was an individual that would give you the shirt right off his back and ask for nothing in return. He loved to help anyone that needed it. He wasn't selfish, and there was no malice in his heart. Then when Manny needed help himself, no one except his family would help him. The fact that he was ignored is not only unbelievable, but it is also just a criminal act. The individuals involved will have to meet their maker, and they will have to justify their acts. I know that God will have his vengeance then, and that they will rot in hell for all eternity, all for the love of money, which, incidentally they can't take with them. After all, like it says in the Bible, vengeance is the Lord's. May God have mercy on their souls!

I would like to add a letter that my mother, Manny's grandmother, wrote to him.

My Dear grandson Manny,

Handsome man, grandson, son, brother and cousin. You were full of love for all of your family. You were a hard worker, very responsible and well educated. Fate gambled with your life and you lost and we your family also lost. God called you home and you had to be with him in paradise. To a place where there is no pain and no hunger or sickness, where everything is love and happiness. I know that you are in a great place where no one can cause you pain. I feel great sorrow in my heart that you had to go so young, but this was part of God's great plan. You came to us and gave us all your love and happiness. When you died you left us with a lot of pain and sadness in our hearts. My only consolation is that I know you are better off with God and all the Saints in Heaven, where you will always be young and healthy. All of your great qualities that were beautiful and made you one of the most honest of men that have walked the earth. You no longer suffer from sickness, pain or hunger. You no longer feel hot or cold and most of all humiliation. You know of the selfishness and greed of man for that cursed paper called money. May God have mercy on those individuals! Every bad thing that is done to us on this earth we leave it to God. My dearest child, my beautiful grandson Manny. May God have mercy for the humiliation and disregard that these damned hospitals, doctors, and nurses showed you. I take solace in the fact that they will for all your pain and they will suffer more than you and we did when judgment day comes. May God bless you and give you shelter in his blessed arms, until we are reunited again.

Until then I give you thanks for giving us all your love and for the decency of loving us. I will love you eternally, Grandma.

My father wrote this for him:

> This Letter is for my grandson Manny . . . Dear Manny, when you first came to our family for some reason I didn't treat you like the grandson or person you really were. Until you taught me to love you more and more. I think back to when I used to visit your home and you used to come to me and say "Grandpa come I want to show you something." Then you would show me a new game or movie or something that you had gotten recently. Oh how I miss that!!! I wish you were here to give me all your love and I could give you all my love. The same way I tried to show Kenneth how much I love him. I know that one day I will see you again. Until then I miss you and love you always. Love, Grandpa.

I would like to clarify that my father in the beginning did not want to get too attached to Manny. He figured that because Levia and I were so young, we were just weren't going to last. He didn't want to have his heart broken in case that were true. But as time went by and Levia and I lasted through the test of time, he got attached to Manny, and he loved his first grandson with all his heart.

There were so many dreams that Manny had. He wanted to get married and have kids. Since he was a chef and his mother was a baker, they wanted to open a bakery together. In fact, they were looking into that possibility in the year before he had gotten sick. These dreams and aspirations were stripped from not only Manny but us as well. Stripped because the health-care professionals (and I use this term with great indifference) decided that Manny's life wasn't worth saving. They stole all his dreams and things that he wanted to accomplish in life. What gave them the right to do this? We will never have grandchildren from him. We will never see the exceptional man that I know he would have been.

Can you believe that this happened here in the USA? Unbelievable, isn't it? But I assure you that this did happen. This story is absolutely true. In the eleven-plus years since his passing, our story has stayed the same. I truly hope that this triggers something in our society to improve our system that doesn't work. It is not fair to everyone. We live by a motto that says, "All men are created equal, equality for all." Then why not in our health-care system?

You might be saying to yourself, "Well, you should have done more to get Manny his care. You should have taken him to Stony Brook Hospital instead." To tell you the truth, we asked ourselves these exact things after Manny had passed. But you know what? He was sent to a hospital that specialized in his type of care. He couldn't have gone to a better place. If, God forbid, you have an AVM, this is where you want to go. They are well equipped to handle these types of maladies. Not only that, he should have been treated. It is as simple as that!

There is no conceivable excuse that could justify how Manny was ignored. No one should be treated this way. How can anyone accept the fact that money is more important than a person's life? This is just, in my opinion, a criminal act; it's murder, given the fact that these doctors claimed that Manny's condition wasn't an emergency, especially since they claimed his AVM was severe. They ran a calculated risk, and Manny lost. Then to casually claim that they weren't responsible is just mind-boggling. They were not only legally but also ethically responsible to treat him after they accepted him as a patient. They blatantly chose to not treat him. They admitted that they were waiting for insurance. They knew the risks; so yes, it was murder. They willfully chose to delay his treatment! You be the judge.

Now I would like to tell you about my younger son, Kenneth. First, because he too had a life-threatening health condition. He was diagnosed with Hodgkin's lymphoma (Hodgkin's disease). This is, as you remember, a cancer of the lymph nodes. It was also stated in

Manny's autopsy that he had nodules in his spleen consistent with Hodgkin's disease. Manny's doctors tried to say that he would have died from this. I want to show you how false this statement is. I also want to show you the difference of the care because Kenneth had health insurance. I also want to show you that even with insurance, Kenneth still had gotten bills for his treatment. Insurance does not pay for everything.

Kenneth was going to need to receive chemotherapy. Do you know how chemotherapy works? You are given poison that is introduced into your body. Since the cancer cells are quick-developing cells, much faster than normal healthy cells, they are able to use this poison. It affects the cancer much quicker than normal cells. So you are filled with enough chemotherapy to literally bring you to the edge of death. Then they stop and let your body slowly recover to start it all over again. Gruesome, isn't it? But this is what we do to treat cancer. Here is his story.

Kenneth was going to college to major in computer gaming. He was in final semester, and he registered to take summer classes. He wasn't able to go, however, because he said he wasn't up to it, so he withdrew from the classes. I was a bit angry at him because I thought he was just being lazy. Little did I know that he had a very good reason for doing this. I'm sorry, Kenneth, for thinking otherwise.

On the week of July 9, 2015, the week of Manny's birthday, we decided to take our RV and go for a camping trip. We all decided to go to Green Point Long Island. When our trip ended, my son, Kenneth, Manny's younger brother, got sick. He had a cough and a fever. I took him to our family doctor. His name is Dr. Tomasso. He has been our family doctor for the better part of sixteen years. It was thought that he had an upper respiratory infection. He gave him antibiotics and a cough suppressant. Kenneth took his medication and got better.

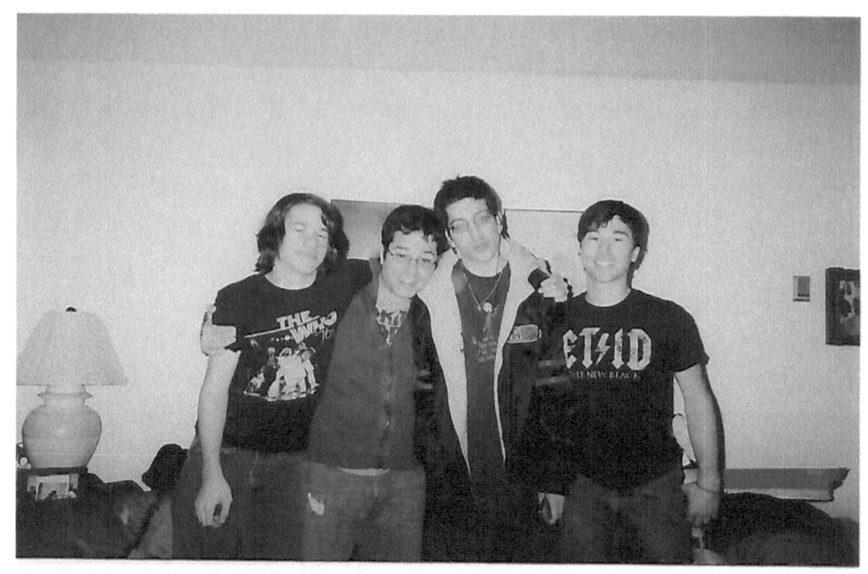

One missing, the cousins together without Manny

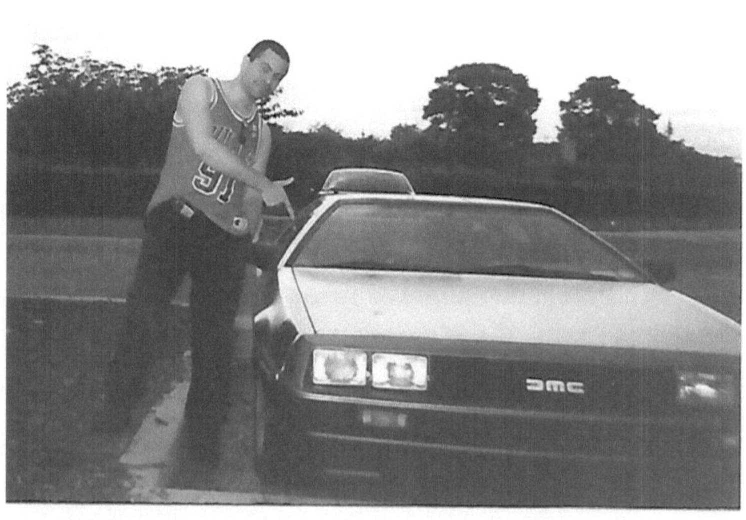

Manny's dream car, dreams that were never fulfilled

Then we decided to take another vacation, and we decided to go upstate for another RV trip. So on the week of August 5, 2015, we took our RV and headed for Oneonta, New York. It was a long five-hour trip from our house. We got off at the Roscoe exit, and I decided to get gas at the local gas station. Unfortunately, I took the turn too sharp and damaged the RV and ended up breaking the hookup pipes. Well, this ended our trip. So we headed back to Long Island.

On the way back, I took the wrong exit and ended up getting lost in Bear Mountain. Finally, I found my way back to the highway and continued on our trek home. I decided to leave our RV at the storage facility. It was about 1:00 a.m., and we unloaded the RV and packed up our suburban and continued home. It was eleven hours from the time we left our house that we arrived back home.

Kenneth, by this time, was complaining that he again wasn't feeling well. He had a relapse. He started coughing again, and he had a fever. I called our doctor, but he was on vacation. So we went to the doctor that was covering for him. She prescribed a different antibiotic and cough medicine. He took his medicine and got better. About a week later, he started coughing again. So on August 24, 2015, he returned to our family doctor. This time he found a lump on his upper chest by the neck area. He was concerned, and he ordered a chest x-ray.

I took him for his x-ray two days later on August 26, 2015. After the x-ray was done, we were told everything was okay but to wait for a digital copy of the x-ray. I suspected something was wrong at this point. Normally, you aren't given a copy of an x-ray unless something is wrong or you asked for it, which we didn't. I took the copy and left, and we went home.

We arrived home, and Kenneth went his room to rest. I wasn't home fifteen minutes when the phone rang. It was our family doctor. He said he had to see Kenneth right away. I knew that something was wrong, just as I suspected. I told Kenneth to get dressed. He had undressed and went back to bed. I informed him that the doctor wanted to see him immediately.

My wife and I decided that Kenneth and I would go and that she would stay home. She was working in the garden. Kenneth got dressed, and less than half hour later, we were at the doctor's office. The waiting room was packed with patients. We checked in and were immediately taken to the back and taken to an examination room. I immediately thought, "Wow, a waiting room full of patients and we are given the red carpet treatment." I said to myself, "This can't be good."

Doctor Tomasso came into the examination room several minutes later, and he started examining Kenneth. He asked Kenneth if he had night sweats. Kenneth answered, "When I was sick and had fever, yes, but not now." He gave Kenneth an extensive checkup, asking Kenneth questions as he examined him. Finally, I asked the doctor, "Is anything wrong?" Then we were finally told that the x-ray came back negative. "I'm glad you are here and not your wife," he said. He was referring to Manny, of course; he knew our whole story. He stated that "Kenneth may have lymphoma or testicular cancer." My world came crashing down. I thought, "Oh no, not again! Oh my God, can't do this again! I can't bury another child!"

You see, Kenneth is twenty-four years old. That was the same age Manny died. I was the one who received the news by Manny's doctor that he had an AVM. Now I am receiving the news that Kenneth might have cancer. When you hear the word *cancer*, you immediately think the worst. I thought, "Oh, God, not him too. You can't take him also." I kept my composure outside even though inside I was a nervous wreck.

Our doctor then gave us referrals for a surgeon to do a biopsy. He also gave us a referral for an oncologist. Then he gave us a copy of the x-ray report. Kenneth and I went home. While I was driving home, I thought, "Oh my God, how do I tell my wife Levia that our son may have cancer?" Kenneth was sort of in shock, as was I. Then Kenneth said, "This can't be cancer. This has to be from the infection that my lymph nodes are swollen." This was a reasonable statement. That could be true, I said, but we must find out for sure. We arrived home, and Kenneth went straight to his room. He looked shocked, annoyed, and sad.

Levia was outside in the yard, doing yard work. I opened the back door and stood on our deck. I looked out to where she was and said, "Come inside."

She answered, "What happened? What's wrong? What did the doctor say?"

I repeated, "Come inside please."

She immediately dropped the garden hose, which she held in her hands, and she came inside. I took a deep breath and said as my voice cracked, "Kenneth has lymphoma."

She replied, "No, that can't be right."

I replied, "That's what the doctor said."

"That can't be right," she said again. "He has a respiratory infection."

"That's what I thought, but apparently not," I said.

I explained to her that we now had to see a surgeon and take him to an oncologist. I will never forget her face after she absorbed the information. "They are wrong. This can't be right. God wouldn't take Kenneth away."

"Maybe they are wrong, but we have to make sure," I said. "We can't just assume that they're wrong, and if he does have cancer, if we don't do anything, he will die."

She agreed with that statement. Then I immediately contacted my job and explained to them the situation I faced and that I will be taking a leave of absence, which they so graciously granted.

Then my wife and I agreed not to tell my parents about the situation yet. After all, it wasn't positive yet that Kenneth had cancer. Why worry them if maybe it's not? I did, however, did tell my sister that lives in North Carolina, who happens to be a doctor in pharmacy and, as luck would have it, specializes in cancer and chemotherapy. After the initial shock, she reassured me that both cancers were curable. Then she explained what to look for and what to expect. I thank God that I have her as a resource. I also told her not to tell our parents; she agreed.

My wife called her mother, but she too was unable to contact her. She finally contacted her sister, and she told her the situation.

Then she informed Levia that her mother was having surgery and that when it was over, she would inform her. Her family was in disbelief.

The rest of that day we all walked around like zombies. We all had feelings of anxiety, anger, disbelief, and several other emotions that I can't even describe. I immediately realized that I had to forget all my emotions and be strong for my family. Easier said than done. So I swallowed my emotions and became a rock even though I was dying inside. So after the initial shock, I made an appointment for Kenneth to see the oncologist and the surgeon.

So as it happened, the surgeon's appointment came first. The day came, and we went to see the surgeon. He checked Kenneth and said he would schedule him to have his biopsy right away. So Kenneth was scheduled for his biopsy the Tuesday after Labor Day. The hospital he was to have it done at was the infamous Brookhaven Hospital, not my hospital of choice. The only reason we reluctantly agreed to take him there was because it was only to be a one-day thing. He would have the operation and leave the same day.

Then the day arrived to see the oncologist. His name is Dr. Syali. We took him to his office in Patchogue, which is a town on Long Island. The name of the facility is North Shore Hematology Oncology Associates (NSHOA). Needless to say, we were nervous. The first thing that was done was they drew blood for a blood test. When the doctor came to see Kenneth, we gave him the x-ray report that we got from our family doctor. He read the report and examined Kenneth. Then the doctor settled down and started to talk to us. He stated that Kenneth most likely have lymphoma, but he may have testicular cancer. Either way, the prognosis was good. He also said there was an outside chance this was caused by his persistent infection. He said he wanted to have a biopsy and to have an ultrasound of the scrotum. We told him that he was already scheduled for the biopsy, which he was pleased to hear. "Then I will order an ultrasound," he said.

He tried to reassure us, stating that both type of cancers are curable. "So let me order some tests and find out what's going on, because right now, it's all speculation. Then we can set up treatment schedule that will cure your son." He then ordered a CAT scan of the neck, chest, abdomen, and groin area. He also ordered an ultrasound and wanted to do a bone marrow biopsy. He asked us if we had any questions. We asked him, "If it is cancer, will he need to have chemotherapy?" He answered yes, then he told us of the possible side effects and what to expect. He also prescribed Kenneth an antibiotic to treat the respiratory infection he had, and stunned as we were, we left.

On the way home, Kenneth said, "You guys set up all the appointments, the transportation to and from, and make all decisions regarding my treatment. I will worry about showing up and getting better. Deal?"

We answered deal. I told him I will be his personal chauffer and take him door to door. I also told him, "Your mother and I will take good care of you no matter what comes."

Levia said, "Yes, we will take care of you and make sure you have all you need to make this as comfortable as possible." When we arrived home, we set up his appointments for his CAT scan and his ultrasound and got his prescription filled.

That evening, Brookhaven Hospital called to tell us to bring Kenneth in for his pretesting. They scheduled it for the Thursday before Labor Day. We set up the time. They explained that Kenneth had to fast. No food or drink after midnight the night before. So we followed the instructions we were given. We went to bed and took him the next day.

I guess here I should add that we were really unaware exactly what the patient and the family go through when cancer becomes part of the equation. Life becomes a series of tests and what seems like endless waiting, which seems like an eternity. Nights of little or no sleep. The endless worry of the situation we faced. We had no idea what we were in for. But we were about to find out.

Levia and I woke up early Thursday morning. We woke Kenneth up and told him to get ready. He got dressed and waited for me to take him for his tests. We got into my Suburban and headed to the hospital. When we arrived, I parked in the parking lot, and we walked to the main entrance. When we got to the front desk, we told the guard that Kenneth was here for pretesting. He told us to sit down and wait until the escort came. He called for an escort, and we sat down. About five minutes later, the escort came and led us to the pre-op testing area. Kenneth was asked for his identification and his insurance card. He gave them to her, and she gave him a clipboard and was asked to fill out the paperwork. I filled out the paperwork, handed it back to the receptionist, and sat down to wait.

Several minutes later, Kenneth's name was called, and we were led to an examination room. We settled in and waited for the nurse to return. A while later, a nurse came in to draw blood. Then I informed her that Kenneth had a blood test a couple of days ago and asked if it was necessary to take blood again. She said she would check, and off she went. When she came back, she asked us if we had a copy of the results. We kept a folder with all of Kenneth's results, but as it turned out, I forgot the paperwork at home. I told her I would go get it, but she said don't bother. She asked us who his doctor was, and we gave her the information. Then she said that she would get the information from the doctor's office.

When she returned, she said she got the information and that Kenneth didn't have to have blood drawn again. This made my son happy, because you see, he tells everyone he's allergic to needles. Then another nurse came in identified herself and started to ask Kenneth a series of questions. She asked about his medical history, questions like if he ever had surgery before, if he was allergic to any medication, if he ever had anesthesia before, family history with cancer, etc., that type of stuff. We answered the questions as best as we could. Then she asked if Kenneth knew what he was having done. He answered, "I'm here to get tested to have a biopsy of my swollen lymph node, to see if in fact I have cancer." After the series of questions was over, she told us to wait for the nurse practitioner.

We waited for a long while, and the practitioner still hadn't come. I was starting to get concerned because I had to take Kenneth for his ultrasound at a facility nearby. So my wife went out to see what was taking so long. She explained that he had another appointment. She was told that the practitioner would be in shortly. Still a while went by and my wife again went to see what the delay was. The nurse asked her if the practitioner had not come to see him yet. My wife answered no. The nurse said, "I will see what the delay is."

As it happens, my wife passed the practitioners' office and heard her talking to another nurse about personal matters.

The practitioner finally came in and started to ask Kenneth questions again, almost the exact same questions that were just asked before. We answered them, and she took his temperature. She checked his blood pressure, checked his swollen lymph node, then told us when to report to the hospital to get the procedure done. We left and I took Kenneth for his ultrasound. We arrived at the facility for the ultrasound. It was the same place he had his chest x-ray done. This was a pretty painless experience. We were in and out. We were there maybe thirty minutes or so.

So we enjoyed the Labor Day weekend. We tried to live life as normal as possible. The weather was nice. We did barbecues. We watched movies at home. I played video games with Kenneth, all in an attempt to keep things as close to normal as we could. But always in the back of my mind was that Kenneth might have cancer. I just couldn't shake that uneasy feeling of dread.

The morning of September 8, 2015, the day after Labor Day had finally arrived. Levia and I woke up super early. We started our day at 6:00 a.m. Levia made coffee, which was the norm for us. We watched our normal Christian programs on TV. We silently said our prayers and started getting ready for what was to come later. I was so nervous that I couldn't keep my mind on any task without drifting off into space.

I woke up Kenneth about 9:00 a.m. I thought that he would give me trouble, but he actually got right up and started his day. He washed up and got dressed, and we all waited for the time to leave. I know that I was nervous; Levia was nervous also. Kenneth seemed to be very calm and cool. He told us to take it easy, that he'd get there, they would knock him out, and when he awoke, it would be over. Imagine that, the one that actually had to go through it was calmer than we were.

At 10:00 a.m. we gathered our things, and I went out and started the car. Several minutes later, Kenneth and my wife came out. They got in the car, and we left. The ride was uneventful; we pretty much didn't say much. My heart was racing faster and faster the closer we got to the hospital. Then finally we arrived. I parked the car, and we went inside.

We arrived at the reception desk, and I told the guard that Kenneth was here for ambulatory surgery. He gave us our passes and told us to take the main elevator to the second floor and then make three lefts and a right. We did as was instructed, and when we arrived, there was a nurse waiting for Kenneth. We were told to wait in the waiting room then while they prepped him, then they would come and get us so we could sit with him in the patient waiting area.

About fifteen minutes later, the nurse returned and took us to the patient waiting area. When we got there, Kenneth had an IV in his arm, and he seemed quite comfortable. We sat with him awhile, then another nurse came in and asked me for my cell phone number to call us when the operation was over, which I gave her. Then the nurse said she was going to take us to the operating room area. Then she told us that we were allowed to go to that area but that we would have to gown up; we agreed. She took the bed over to the OR area, which was close by. She gave my wife and me a disposable, gown along with shoe covers and a cap.

While we were waiting, the OR nurse came in and identified himself. He asked Kenneth a series of questions, which Kenneth answered. He asked Kenneth to sign some papers, and Kenneth signed them. Then the nurse said the anesthesiologist would be coming to talk to him, as well as the surgeon. Then he asked if we had any questions. We said no, and then he left. We stayed there watching the movie *Tom Thumb*, which was playing on the TV that was just above us on the wall.

A short time later, the anesthesiologist came in and asked Kenneth another series of questions, which Kenneth answered. He asked if Kenneth was allergic to anything. Kenneth answered, "Yes, cheap orange soda." The doctor chuckled. Then he asked if he ever had any anesthesia. Kenneth said no. Then he explained what he was going to do. Kenneth said, "That's fine, as long as you knock me out." The anesthesiologist chuckled again and then asked Kenneth to sign a consent form authorizing him to give Kenneth anesthesia. Kenneth signed the paper. He asked if there were any questions. Kenneth said no and he left.

A short time later, the surgeon came in. He also asked Kenneth a series of questions and marked the area where Kenneth was to have the incision made. He told us the risks associated with the surgery. Then he asked us if we had any questions. We said that we didn't, then he told Kenneth, "I'll see you inside," and he left. We waited a short time, then the OR nurse came and took Kenneth into the operating room, and we were told to wait in the waiting room outside. We took off all the surgical stuff and left.

We went out into the waiting room and nervously waited. I brought a book to read to pass the time. I tried to read it, but I can't tell you how many times I kept reading the same page over and over. No matter how many times I read the page, it didn't make any sense. My mind was on Kenneth. Like any parent, I was worried. Every minute felt like an hour; it felt like time was at a standstill.

Then my wife and I decided to go to the coffee shop to grab a bite to eat. We went downstairs and entered the coffee shop. We got a cup of coffee, and we split a turkey wrap between us. The coffee was pretty good, and the wrap was fresh. We ate it, drank our coffee, and sat there waiting.

Finally, my cell phone rang; it was the surgeon. He told me that Kenneth's procedure was over. Everything went well, and he was in the recovery room. He then told me that he wanted to see Kenneth in a week. He told me not to worry about the bandages, that he would remove them. He said Kenneth could shower after two days but to keep the area dry. He also said that he would give Kenneth a pain killer, and he gave me verbal instructions about how he should take them.

We left the coffee shop and went upstairs. We returned to the waiting room. About a half hour later, a nurse came and got us and took us to Kenneth. To my surprise, Kenneth was awake and alert. He was eating a snack and drinking apple juice that he was given. I asked him how he felt. Kenneth answered, "I feel pretty good." My wife and I were relieved. The nurse checked his blood pressure and took his temperature, which was normal. She gave us the prescription for his pain killer; she also gave us his discharge instructions. Then she told me to get the car and wait by the front entrance. About ten minutes later, Kenneth was brought out in a wheelchair. He got into the car, and we went home.

Kenneth had an appointment the next day for a bone marrow biopsy. My wife and I cancelled it because we thought it was best to wait for the results of this biopsy. We didn't want him to suffer two procedures back to back. We were thinking optimistically. We thought maybe this biopsy would come back negative. We were told it took a week to ten days to get the results.

On Friday, September 11, 2015, a date that has a new meaning for my family, Kenneth's oncologist called and asked us why we cancelled the bone marrow biopsy. We explained that Kenneth was still sore and we thought it best to wait for the results of the biopsy. I told him, "Why subject Kenneth to an evasive procedure unless we are sure he had cancer? Then he broke the news. He stated that he spoke to the pathologist and told me that Kenneth did in fact have lymphoma. Kenneth had Hodgkin's lymphoma. My world came crashing down. My fears were now a reality. We made the appointment for his bone marrow biopsy. I hung up the phone, feeling numb with a feeling of disbelief.

My mind started racing, trying to absorb this bad news. I wondered how this could be happening. Kenneth never smoked, he never took drugs, he lived a clean life. He did everything that was expected of him, and this was his reward. My emotions were running wild. It was like a ton of bricks were just dropped on my lap. Cancer! I thought the worst. Oh my God, Kenneth is gravely ill. I wanted to crawl under a rock and die. I had a mixture of anger, sadness, anxiety, sorrow, and other emotions that have no words to describe.

The time came to break the news to Kenneth. He was in his room, sleeping, or so I thought. We were in the office, which was Manny's bedroom. This room was opposite Kenneth's room. Since we were talking to the doctor on speaker phone, he overheard the conversation. Levia and I went to his room to tell him. He was in his bed. I went to speak, and he told us, "Get out of here and leave me alone." I didn't know that he knew the outcome of the conversation with the doctor. I said, "Kenneth, it's official. You have lymphoma. You need to have a bone marrow biopsy." He was angry and said, "I know, I heard. Just get the hell out of my room and leave me alone." We tried to tell him he wasn't alone in an attempt to comfort him. He just had so much anger that no matter what we said, it made no difference. So we respected his wishes and left him alone. I can only imagine what he was feeling. I know how I felt, but I wasn't the one who had cancer; he was. The rest of the day passed, and we were like zombies going through the motions but feeling lifeless, with no meaning.

I broke the news to my sister; she got upset. She kept trying to reassure me that Hodgkin's disease was very curable. I listened to her, but it was like being in a tunnel and words were like echoes. I told her that I had to tell our parents, who, as you know, did not know. She asked me if I wanted her to tell them. I said, "No, I'll do it." Of course, that was easier said than done.

I called my parents' house, and my mother answered the phone. She said, "Hi, how are you guys?"

I said I was okay, but she immediately sensed something was wrong.

She asked, "What's the matter? What's wrong?"

I answered, "It's Kenneth."

Her voice went from cheerful to one of concern. "What's wrong," she asked.

"He has lymphoma." My voice cracked as I said it.

My mother lost it. She got hysterical and started crying. My father, who was evidently near her, asked her what was wrong. She told him Kenneth had lymphoma. He took the phone from her and asked me what had happened. I told him that Kenneth had lymphoma. He wasn't sure what lymphoma was, and he asked what it was. I told him that it was cancer of the lymph nodes. He asked many questions, and I answered them as best as I could. Then he said, "We will see you later. We are coming over."

A short time later, my parents arrived. My mother came to me, and I lost it. I hugged her and broke into tears. "Kenneth has cancer," I said.

She comforted me as best as she could. I then composed myself and held back my emotions. I kissed my old man, who was looking quite distraught, with teary eyes. In fact, we were all teary eyed. They went in to see Kenneth, who was still in his room. They spoke to him briefly and tried to reassure him. He was still angry, not at them of course, but at the situation he faced. He told them that he wanted to be left alone. So we left him alone and left his room. Kenneth's emotions were justified, of course. He lost his brother at the same age he was.

We went to the kitchen table, and we sat down. I made coffee, and we drank and talked about the prospects and what was to be done next. We chatted for a while, but to be quite honest, no matter what was said, the fact that Kenneth had cancer was on all our minds. That damn word *cancer* brings nothing but the worst thoughts imaginable. They stayed for a while and then left.

The next day we went to the oncologist's office to have the bone marrow biopsy done. They drew blood from Kenneth, and then we were taken to an examination room. A nurse came and took his temperature and his blood pressure. Then she explained what was going to be done. We asked some questions that were answered. Then she said, "Wait here until the person comes to do the procedure, but you can't be present when the procedure is started."

A short time later, we were asked to leave, and we went out into the waiting room. We waited until we were asked to return and sit with Kenneth to see the doctor. We asked Kenneth how it went. Kenneth said, "It hurt like hell. I felt a crunch as the needle went through my bone."

The doctor came in a short time later and explained to us in more detail what was coming next and what course of treatment was best for Kenneth. He told us that Kenneth was to go through six cycles of chemotherapy over a six-month period. He explained that two infusions equaled one cycle. He was to be given four different types of chemo back to back. Each infusion was to be given every other week, with an office visit every week in between. He explained that many tests still remained to be done to see how far the cancer had progressed.

Kenneth was to have a CAT scan done the following week. He already had his ultrasound done. Then the doctor told us that Kenneth needed an echocardiogram done, that he needed to see a lung specialist, because one of the chemo drugs he was going to get could affect the lungs and could cause lung damage. He wanted to get a baseline on Kenneth's lung function prior to any chemo being given. He gave us a referral for the lung doctor, with the address and name of the doctor.

He also wanted to have an MRI of the brain because Manny had died from an AVM and he wanted to make sure Kenneth didn't have the same condition. Then he ordered Kenneth to have a PET scan, which is similar to a CAT scan, only that it is more precise in evaluating cancer. He also wanted to have a port implanted so that the chemo would be administered through the port rather than on a vein in his arm. The chemo drugs could collapse the veins in his arms, making it difficult to receive treatment. He said that he would take care of all the prior approvals and he would schedule us to see the educator that was part of the treatment. She would explain the side effects on all the different chemo he would be getting. He also wanted Kenneth to do sperm banking. He explained that chemo can make him sterile. So he wanted Kenneth to freeze his sperm for the future.

We set all his appointments as the preapprovals came. Kenneth had all his tests done one right after the other. The MRI was pretty painless. All Kenneth had to do was lie on a table and stay absolutely still. That was simple enough for Kenneth to do. Then he would go into a tunnel that uses a large electromagnet to take readings of his skull. The procedure takes a while, and it was necessary to have this done. We wanted to know if Kenneth had what his brother had. I prayed silently, hoping for the best.

The test was done, and we left. Then Kenneth had to have a PET scan done. This required Kenneth to fast for at least six hours before the procedure was done. He also had to follow a low-carb high-protein diet. He wasn't allowed to have sugar either. He wasn't allowed bread, pasta, or any other grain products. He couldn't have any fruits or any soda or any drink that contained sugar. He was allowed to eat meats such as chicken, fish, and beef. Vegetables were good, and he was to drink plenty of water. So he did as he was told, and he was ready for the PET scan.

Kenneth had to arrive on time because the PET scan requires that you get a radioactive isotope that is given intravenously. This of course was something Kenneth wasn't looking forward to. Remember that Kenneth is allergic to needles according to him. LOL! Then he has to wait an hour before the PET scan could be done. Well, he went through it, and he was done with it. He really hated having this done, but he had to get it done. They needed to see how much of his lymphatic system was affected.

We then went to see the nurse educator. She explained which chemo drugs he was getting and the side effects associated to each. He was to have a treatment known as ABVD. This is the first-line treatment given to lymphoma patients, and it is supposed to be very effective. He was to receive Adriamycin (A) and was supposed to be given as a push. That means that it is to be given in a syringe and administered directly into his IV line. Then he was to be given bleomycin (B), and that one is mixed in an IV bag and then it is infused via the IV line slowly. This incidentally is the chemo that is known to damage the lungs. Then he was to get vinblastine (V); this was also to be administered as a push. Then finally he was to be given dacarbazine (D), which is given as another IV bag or infusion.

She explained all the different side effects of each, mostly nausea, fatigue, mouth sores, loss of hair, sensitivity to the sun, just to name a few. Then she told us about how he was going to be given antinausea medicine to alleviate the sense of nausea. She was very thorough in telling us about every possible aspect of getting chemotherapy, which by the way sounded awful, and poor Kenneth was listening to all this. I felt sorry for him. He looked like he was in shock. She asked us if we had questions. We had several, which she very professionally answered. Then after we were educated about it all, we left. Deep inside we really didn't want Kenneth to go through any more suffering, but what choice did we have?

I called the lung doctors' office that was recommended to make his appointment and was told that the earliest that Kenneth could be seen was in mid-October. I told them that he needed to have this done sooner because he had cancer and needed to get chemo right away. Sorry, she said, but that was the best she could do. We called the oncologist's office and explained the situation to them. That was unacceptable, they said and told us not worry, that they would take care of it, which they did. We were given a date and time to see the lung doctor. I still don't understand how when I called there was no appointment available, but when the oncologist's office called, the appointment was made for the next day.

We took Kenneth to see the lung doctor. He had his pulmonary function test done. The test required Kenneth to blow into a machine that measures how much air goes in and out of the lungs. It also measures the amount of oxygen that is absorbed through the lungs. This requires different types of breathing into the machine. In one test you breathe normally, nothing unusual there. In another one he had to inhale deeply, taking as much air as was physically possible, then he had to blow hard and keep blowing until the tech told him to stop. Then another test required Kenneth to pant like a dog or like he was hyperventilating. Then the tests end, and all information are recorded on different graphs and line, each representing a specific thing.

Then we were taken to the examination room and waited for the doctor. He came in and identified himself. He checked out all the info that was recorded on the charts. Then he checked his heart, listened to his lungs, and of course, he took his pulse, temperature, and blood pressure. Then after the exam was completed, he sat down with us and told us Kenneth's lungs were in excellent condition and that he was able to start receiving his chemotherapy. Then he said that this test was to get a baseline for the function of his lungs. Then he said that he was going to get several of these tests throughout his chemotherapy, to see if there was any degradation of the function of his lungs. That would determine if he could receive his bleomycin.

My wife and I prepped Kenneth's room to make it ready for a chemotherapy patient. We got him a mini refrigerator for his room. We stocked it with drinks, Jell-O, puddings, yogurts, and such. We stocked his room with snacks and other things that we could think of.

This way Kenneth had anything he needed right there at his room. We were determined to make things as comfortable as possible for him.

Then we had to see the surgeon for his check up and to remove Kenneth's bandages. He examined Kenneth and was pleased with the way the wound looked. Then he told us that Dr. Syali had asked him to put a port in Kenneth's chest. He told us that it was to be an ambulatory surgery, which made Kenneth happy. He explained what a port was and how it was placed into the chest and was attached to a vein near the neck. He told us about the risks involved and asked us if we had questions, which we didn't. He made the appointment for the surgery and told us we would get a call from the hospital to set up his preop testing. He told us he'd see us soon on the day of the surgery, and we left.

The hospital called, and we took Kenneth for his testing. The experience was pretty much like the last time, except we didn't have to wait for the nurse practitioner this time. Then the day came for his surgery. We arrived and made the three lefts and a right. He was again taken to the waiting area, and he was prepped for surgery. We then went to the waiting area when the time came. The OR nurse came then the anesthesiologist then the surgeon, one right after another, just like the last time. The appropriate questions were asked, the papers were signed, and the area was marked. Then he was off to have the surgery. About an hour later, it was over. Everything went well, and he went to the recovery room.

The doctor gave me instructions again. He prescribed more pain killers for Kenneth. He again wanted to see Kenneth a week later. We were taken into the recovery room, and again Kenneth was alert and eating snacks. We asked him how he felt. He told us he felt fine. He was actually in good spirits. The nurse took his vitals, and when he was ready to be discharged, we were given instructions about bathing and taking his pain killer. She gave us his prescription, and I went to get the car to meet them at the front entrance.

About ten minutes later, Kenneth arrived, and we went home. Kenneth then had to see the surgeon again for his postop checkup a week later. The surgeon came and took off his bandages, and he was pleased with the way the wound looked. "I do good work," he said. He did actually. Kenneth's scars looked good and, by the way, healed nicely. He told us that it was okay to start using the port. Then he wished Kenneth good luck with the chemotherapy. "I hope all goes well for you." We thanked him, and we left.

We went to see the oncologist on his next scheduled appointment. He went over all the results with us. He said that the cancer wasn't in his bone marrow, which was great news. He said his heart and lungs were in great condition, again great news. We didn't say anything about knowing this information from the pulmonologist. He said that the results of the MRI were good. Kenneth did not have any AVMs or aneurisms. My wife and I gave a sigh of relief. He said that the PET scan showed that the lymph node nodules got a little larger. This meant that the swelling got worse since he was first diagnosed.

Then he told us Kenneth had stage four Hodgkin's Lymphoma. Cancer is graded in stages one through four. Stage one is an early stage. Stage four is advanced or severe stage. We explained to the doctor that Kenneth refused to go for the sperm banking. He also tried to change Kenneth's mind, but he refused to budge. He wanted to start his chemo ASAP. So he was scheduled to start chemo on October 2, 2015, the day before his twenty-fifth birthday. "Happy birthday," I thought but kept it to myself.

We went on the rest of the week, trying to live life normally. I spent my days playing video games with Kenneth, trying not to think of Friday, chemo day. We enjoyed ourselves and spent precious moments laughing and joking. We watched movies and played games. We tried to cater to Kenneth because we knew that he was going to have chemo and we knew that it wasn't going to be pleasant for him. It wasn't going to be pleasant for us either, for that matter. Levia started baking cookies and cake for the entire staff. This was something she did every chemo day, which was our way of saying thanks for taking care of Kenneth. Then Thursday came, and we continued to play and spend time together. Then it was time to go to sleep. I couldn't sleep a wink that night; neither could Levia. What parent could?

The next day came, and I woke up Kenneth. I asked him how he slept. He answered surprisingly, "I slept well." "Thank God," I said. He had a light breakfast. Then Levia and I decided that I would accompany Kenneth to the infusion center and that she would stay home. There was no reason for her to witness Kenneth taking chemo; she's been through enough. So it was decided that I would be his infusion buddy. I got to be strong, I thought, but I was extremely nervous. Surprisingly, Kenneth was as cool as a cucumber. He was looking forward to starting his chemo. "Now finally I'm going to kill this damn cancer." Kenneth definitely had the right attitude.

I, on the other hand, was running around like a chicken without a head. It seemed to me like I was wandering around the house not knowing what I was doing. Levia was preparing snacks and drinks for us, so she packed a small cooler that was to become part of our ritual when we went to the cancer clinic. I made sure I had Kenneth's anti-nausea medicine with me. I was supposed to give it to him one hour before he was to get his chemo. I really didn't know what to bring because I've never done this before. I kept wondering what I was forgetting. You know how you get that nagging feeling that you forgot something. Thank God I didn't forget a thing. When the time came, I got the car ready, and off we went.

So Kenneth and I went to the infusion center. We went to the infusion area and were told to pick a seat anywhere. Kenneth sat down on a recliner, and I took a stool and sat at his feet. His temperature and blood pressure were taken, then he was weighed. The nurse immediately came and drew his blood. A short time later, the nurse hung a bag of normal saline. The pharmacist came and asked if we were told that he needed something cold, like ice or a Slurpee, to freeze his mouth while they were infusing the first chemo. We told him we didn't know this. He answered, "Don't worry. You have time to go to 7-Eleven." I gave Kenneth his antinausea capsule that he had to take one hour prior to the start of chemo and left to get his Slurpee. My wife called while I was at 7-Eleven, and I told her what was happening so far.

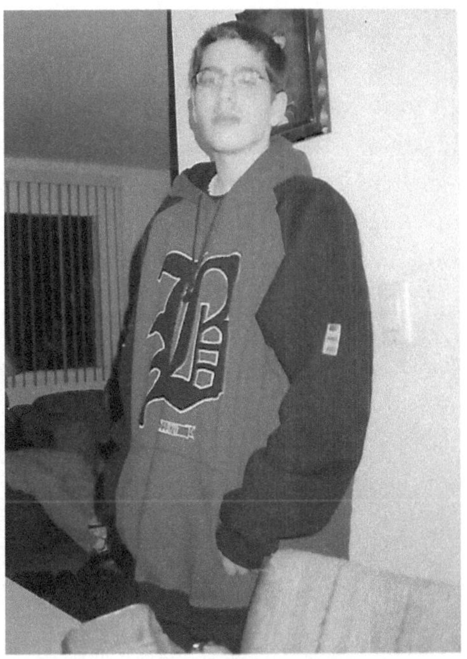

Kenneth Pre-chemo he is wearing one of Manny's hoody's

I returned from 7-Eleven with the Slurpee and handed it to Kenneth. I arrived just in time. The pharmacist had mixed his first chemo. About ten minutes later, the nurse came and started his first dose of chemo. Kenneth started to drink his Slurpee as she pushed the chemo from the syringe into his IV line. Finally it was done; he had received his first of four chemos he was to receive. Immediately after, he received the second chemo; this one was given through a small IV bag. A short time later, that one ended.

So far Kenneth was taking his poison and showed no signs of nausea. I thanked God that he was taking it well. Then the third chemo arrived, and this was also a push. The nurse slowly pushed the chemo into his body until all of it was administered. Kenneth still showed no signs of any nausea. Again I thanked God that he was taking it well. Then the fourth chemo, which was another IV bag, larger than the second one, was infused into the IV line. This one lasted about an hour, and Kenneth again had no nausea.

Kenneth had received all four doses, and he took it well. They hydrated him with the remainder of the normal saline from the IV bag. This lasted about another hour or so, and finally he was done. He had taken his doses, and all went well, no nausea or any other side effects. We gathered our belongings, and I asked Kenneth how he felt, and he answered, "I feel pretty good."

"Thank God," I said. We thanked everyone, and we left.

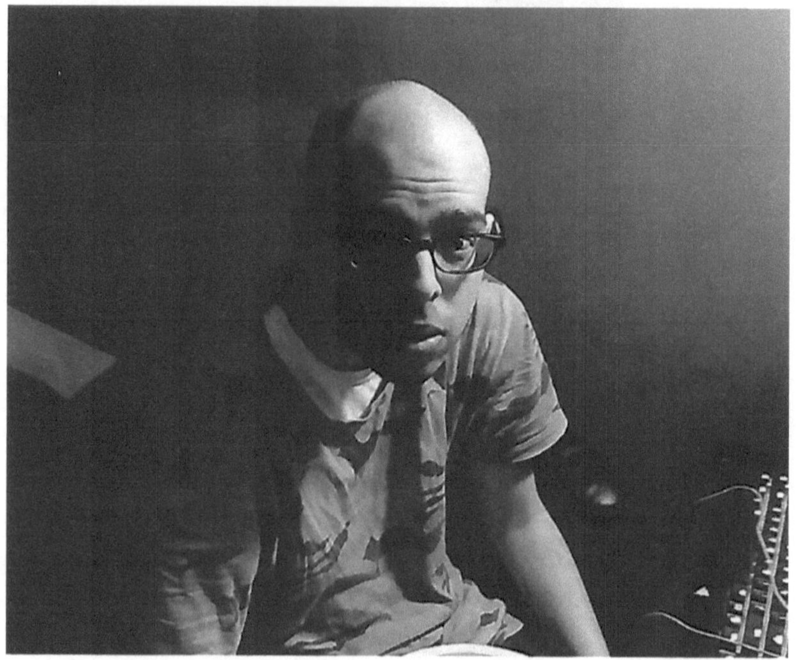

Kenneth post chemo

We arrived home and were greeted by Levia, who was nervously waiting at home. She asked Kenneth how he felt, and he said "I feel good."

"Thank God," she said.

He went to his room, which was now sanitized, because my wife had sterilized it. She cleaned his room and changed all his sheets and pillowcases. She had mopped and wiped all the surfaces with a disinfectant. She did this to make sure Kenneth's environment was free from germs.

You see, when a person receives chemo, his or her immune system bottoms out, making the person susceptible to sickness. This makes the person literally fragile and prone to get sick. So my wife gave Kenneth an environment that was practically germ-free. My wife keeps a clean house, but she wanted to go the extra mile to make sure he was in a sterilized environment.

Kenneth settled down and went straight to bed. I asked him how he felt; he said he was worn out. I didn't wonder why. After all, he was just pumped full of poison. It doesn't cease to amaze me how poison is used to cure cancer. There has to be a better way. It is my opinion that since we have a "for profit" health-care system, and since chemotherapy is so expensive and there is so much money to be made, I believe we will never see a cure other than this aggressive therapy. There is just too much profit to be made, so we keep the status quo. What a shame, and shame on us for allowing it!

So ended his first chemotherapy treatment. I thanked God that it went pretty well. He didn't get nauseous, but there was always the threat to get delayed nausea. So my wife and I slept on the couch for the next couple of days to keep a sharp eye on him so that he wouldn't suffer. He ate and drank for the rest of the day. Kenneth was worn out though. He slept on and off, and I gave him his anti-nausea medicine when they were due. The first night went relatively trouble-free.

The next day also went relatively trouble-free. Life was pretty much normal, as normal as could be anyway. The second and third day went well also. The fourth day, Tuesday, went well. Kenneth ate and drank and took his meds. That night we decided to eat pizza for dinner. Kenneth ate his pizza and drank lemonade. We played video games together to keep his mind off things. After several hours, he got hungry again, and he had the two remaining slices of pizza. Little did we realize we made a big mistake.

The next day, when I awoke, I went to his room and asked him how he felt. Kenneth answered that he had sores in his mouth and that he was in pain. This happened because he ate pizza and the pizza sauce is acidic. He also drank lots of lemonade, also very acidic. Between the two and the fact that chemo can cause mouth sores, he suffered the next few days. He couldn't eat; he couldn't drink without causing pain. This was the first time we were experiencing this. We were naive and had no idea that the pizza and lemonade were going to affect him in this way. Now we know better.

His doctor prescribed something called miracle mouthwash, which helped him temporarily. I got him Cepacol lozenges, which has an anesthetic in it that also made things better for him. The problem was that Kenneth couldn't drink or eat properly, so he got dehydrated. I had to take him in for hydration. Finally, after three grueling days, his sore got better and life got better.

He went to see his oncologist a week after chemo; they checked his blood levels. His white blood cell count was extremely low. His doctor prescribed an antibiotic to prevent him from getting sick. This antibiotic would become part of his daily regimen because he had to take two a day until he was told not to do so any longer. The days went by, and he felt better and better, just in time to fill him with poison again.

The morning of October 16, 2015, arrived. This was the day of his second round of chemotherapy. This would be the end of his first cycle. Kenneth was feeling like himself again. He woke up in good spirits, and we got ready to go to the infusion center. Since everything went well the first time, we weren't as nervous as the last time. Little did we know of what was to come.

We arrived at the infusion center, and everything was done as the last time. They took his blood count. They took his blood pressure, checked his temperature, and his weight was taken. The nurse attached his bag of normal saline via his port. His chemo was a go. I gave him his anti-nausea medicine and went to 7-Eleven to get his Slurpee. When I got back, he started receiving his treatment. The first chemo went in trouble-free. The second also was trouble-free. The third and fourth went in what seemed to be trouble-free. All the while Kenneth ate a doughnut; he had cereal, and everything went fine.

After all the chemo went in and he was being hydrated, Kenneth said, "I'm feeling kind of nauseous." The nurse came and ran to get him a "barf" bag. No sooner did he put it in his hands when out came all he had eaten. Kenneth was vomiting violently. This was heart-wrenching to watch. I felt helpless; there was nothing I could do to help him. Another nurse came with several "barf" bags and handed them to me.

Meanwhile, another nurse came with an IV form of anti-nausea medicine and immediately attached it to his IV line. Kenneth continued vomiting violently. He now had nothing left in his stomach; he had the dry heaves. I have to tell you, this was hard to see. All I could do was hold the bags and stroke his head in a futile attempt to relieve him. Inside I was crying. I was desperately trying to do what I could to comfort him. I felt like I was trying to put out a barn fire with a water pistol. I felt utterly useless.

I said a little prayer for Kenneth, asking God to help him and to give me strength. A short time later, a woman that was the wife of another patient receiving treatment put her attention to Kenneth. She asked me if he was my son. I answered yes. She said, "My god, so young." Then she said, "If you don't mind me asking, what is he here for?"

I answered, "He has Hodgkin's lymphoma."

Then she said she felt for me because she had lost her son, and she understood what it was to see a child suffer.

I immediately thought, "My God, you sent me an angel, someone that understands what I am going through." I had trouble keeping up my composure, to be strong for Kenneth. Then after I prayed, along came this compassionate woman that understood my grief, someone to comfort me in my hour of need. This woman gave me the strength to endure to make me strong. I no longer felt like I was about to lose it.

I told her that I had already lost my first one. This is my second one, and they were both the same age when we found out they were sick. She then told me, "Your first one is in a better place."

I answered, "I know."

In the meantime, Kenneth was still in distress. The nurse came with another anti-nausea IV bag, a different medication. She removed the first one, which was now empty, and replaced it with the new one. Kenneth's distress continued while the IV dripped into his vein. I continued to try to comfort Kenneth.

The woman told me of her experience with her son. I told her about Manny. I told her he died because he had no insurance and was left to die. Our conversation went on for a short time, while Kenneth was still in distress with the dry heaves. All the while, this lovely woman kept giving me the strength I needed to keep my composure.

The IV emptied, and Kenneth was still in distress. Let me tell you, this was heartbreaking. Kenneth didn't seem to be getting any better. Now the nurses, the doctor, and the pharmacist were frantically trying to stop Kenneth's distress. My sister that I was in constant contact with kept texting me, giving suggestions as what to try next as far as controlling the nausea. The staff at the infusion center was on the ball. No sooner did I receive a suggestion when a nurse would come and administer just what my sister suggested and then some. They threw the book at him, so to speak. Nothing seemed to be working, and Kenneth was still in distress. Minutes felt like hours, and all I could do was try to comfort him.

Then this glorious woman—and I am sorry I keep calling her woman because I didn't get her name—said to me, "If you don't mind me asking, do you have any religious beliefs?"

I said, "Yes, I'm a born-again Christian."

Then she said, "Would you mind if I said a prayer for Kenneth?"

"Of course not, please do," I replied.

Then she placed her hand on Kenneth's leg and said a prayer asking God to relieve Kenneth's pain and to cure him of his illness. She also prayed to give me strength and help me with my pain. At the end, Kenneth and I said amen. A very short time later, Kenneth stopped vomiting. By this time, her husband was done with his treatment, and we said our good-byes. I would like to thank this woman for doing what she did. I want her to know that God sent her to be my strength and be our angel at our time of need. God bless you. We will never forget you!

Kenneth was actually feeling better. I thanked God. They hung another bag of normal saline to rehydrate him. About an hour later, the bag emptied, and Kenneth was told he could go home. Before we left, the pharmacist came and promised Kenneth that the next time would be better; we would try a different approach. This was the end of his second treatment. The first cycle was over. It was an experience that Kenneth and I will never forget. Two doses down, ten more to go. At this point, it was not a good prospect. Aside from Manny dying and having to bury him, this was the worst experience of my life. I don't wish this on anyone.

Kenneth seemed to be developing a pattern. He would go get pumped full of poison. He would feel lousy for three days. Then gradually start to feel better day by day. By the time a week went by, he started feeling like himself again. Then he would enjoy the second week feeling great. Unfortunately, this was just in time to start the cycle over again. I got to say, he was taking his dilemma well.

One day I was looking through my e-mail, when I came across the worst news I could receive aside from my son getting sick. My health insurance, Healthcare Republic of New York, was going out of business. They were winding down their operations, they said. My insurance would end January 1, 2016. They would not be issuing renewal policies. This was not the news I wanted to read, not at this point.

Up to this point, the insurance pretty much covered everything. We were only paying our usual copays. Up to this point, we didn't pay for any chemo drugs. Everything went smoothly. I was pleased with my insurance. Now I wondered what would happen. Little did I know I was about to find out.

When my son was diagnosed with cancer, we went to the oncologist that my primary doctor, Dr. Anthony Tomasso, recommended. So we went to see Dr. Gurmohan Syali. He seemed to be a caring, well spoken, and very knowledgeable doctor. To be honest, we wanted to take our son to Memorial Sloan Kettering. But we felt comfortable with Dr. Syali. He was affiliated with North Shore Hematology Oncology Associates (NSHOA). Their motto is "Conquering cancer close to home." So we decided to take him there, mostly because we liked Dr. Syali.

The week of his third chemo treatment, things started to change. We received a call from a pharmacy, one that I never heard of. The pharmacist said she was from Acaria Health and wanted to speak to Kenneth. I told her I was his father, and I asked what this was about. She said she couldn't talk to me and again asked to speak to Kenneth. I told her that I was his health-care proxy and I made all the decisions about his care.

"I have to hear that from the patient," she said.

With that comment, I went to Kenneth's room and told him to tell this person that it was okay to speak to me concerning his care. He told her that his father took care of all aspects of his heath care and directed her to speak to me.

I got back on the phone, and she told me that Dr. Syali ordered Aloxi for Kenneth's next round of chemo. Then I was told that I had to pay sixty dollars, or he wouldn't get his medicine. I answered, "Who are you, and why are you calling demanding money?"

She answered that they were a pharmacy that dealt with NSHOA and that the supplied them with drugs that they normally didn't carry. This kind of caught me off guard, and so I pulled out my visa card and paid for it.

My wife got upset and wanted to know why I paid for the medicine. I explained to her that I was told to pay, or Kenneth would not get his medicine. I knew that Aloxi was an anti-nausea medicine and that we were going to try this at his next chemo treatment. I told her I didn't want to see Kenneth suffer with nausea and vomiting ever again. She was upset with me because she said that NSHOA should supply this. I agreed with her, but I was backed into a corner, and so I paid for it.

A couple of days later, that same pharmacy called again. This time my wife answered the phone. The person asked to speak to Kenneth, and she went to give the phone to Kenneth. You see, she thought it was a nurse that the insurance provided to see how Kenneth was doing. She had no idea that it was the pharmacy again. When Kenneth talked to this person, he was told that they were supplying his chemo and that he had to pay $177 in order to get it, or they wouldn't supply it. My wife told me that his expression changed to one of concern. He told the pharmacist, "Talk to my mom. I don't have anything to do with that."

My wife took the phone again and was told to pay, or he wouldn't get his chemo. Levia said, "Since when do we have to pay? We didn't have to pay the first two times. Why do we have to pay now?"

The pharmacist answered she didn't know why, but we had to pay now. My wife got furious and said, "Oh hell no, I have to look into this." With that she took down the number and the name of the pharmacist. "I'll call you back," she said hung up the phone.

My wife immediately called NSHOA. She was finally got in contact with a person called Michael; he was someone from billing. She explained to my wife that as of October 1, they would no longer be accepting our health insurance because they were going out of business. But we were covered till January 1, he said. Even so, he said the decision was made to no longer accept it. Then she told him, if this decision was made on October 1, why were we not told? She told him he didn't start his chemo till October second, the day after. He didn't have much to say after that statement. Then she said, "If we had known, we would have taken him to Memorial Sloan Kettering." Then she told him that she was going to transfer him to Sloan Kettering.

He answered, "That's not a good idea because that would delay his treatment. He needs to keep his current course of treatment without delay in order to get a positive outcome."

Needless to say, my wife was upset and told him, "I'll call back." My wife called me and told me of the situation. I of course got upset. I asked her why. We didn't pay before. Why now? Then I told her to call Sloan Kettering and explain the situation and see if we could go there instead.

So my wife called Sloan Kettering to inquire about transferring Kenneth to their facility. She explained the situation to them. She was told that what they were doing was unethical. If they accepted his insurance, they were committed to taking care of Kenneth. She was told not to pay for the chemo because they should have the drugs on-site. Then he said if they don't have it on-site, then they shouldn't be in the cancer treatment business. Also he stated that if they refused treatment after the fact, they were liable and faced a huge lawsuit.

Then he explained what had to be done in order to take Kenneth to their facility. She was told to fax all his test results, along with the treatment summary, and to send a copy of his picture identification and a copy of his insurance card. She gathered all she could, because we kept a copy of all his results. The only thing we didn't have was the summary of his last treatment.

When I got home, she explained what she was told by Sloan Kettering. She told me if I had had any questions, to call the number and the extension and talk to them. I called and asked several questions. Then I was told that Kenneth could not be transferred there until they did a second PET scan to see if the treatment was working. "Great," I said, "so we are stuck with them until they complete the third cycle or until after the sixth chemo treatment." With that I didn't bother sending anything because nothing could be done just yet.

So here we were. What could we do but stay and deal with a facility that seemed to care for Kenneth until his health insurance became an issue? Now they didn't seem to care about anything but money. Then again I do understand that chemotherapy is expensive. Dr. Syali, however, didn't care about the insurance issue; he was a man of honor and integrity. He was going to treat Kenneth regardless. That is the problem with the for-profit health-care system that we have in this country. We Americans have to wake up and demand for universal health-care system in this country. This way, everyone involved gets paid. Why not? The rest of the world has it, and it works. But we are conditioned to believe that it won't work because our politicians say it won't, and we as a society drink the Kool-Aid and believe this nonsense.

We don't find cures in this country anymore. We find treatments for illnesses so that big pharmaceutical companies can make a fortune on. They start you on a drug that you have to take indefinitely. Don't get me wrong, I believe in making a profit for businesses or invented products. I don't believe that profit should be made off people's misfortune and especially not in our health-care system. I believe we should try to find cures for illnesses, not find only treatments. This will not happen as long as we have a "for profit" system.

I took him for his third treatment, and he went through it pretty well. The new nausea drugs seemed to work well. After the treatment, Kenneth complained that he was worn out. He spent the next three days sleeping most of the time. Poor kid was truly worn out. I could see it in his expressions. Then finally slowly he recovered from the poison that he was given.

By this time, Kenneth started losing his hair. It was literally coming out on chunks. Kenneth got tired of seeing chunks of hair on his pillow. He went over to Levia and asked her to buzz his hair. "I'm shedding like a cat," he said. My wife kept trying to put it off. She didn't want to buzz his hair off. Then finally Kenneth and I convinced her to do it. She got the buzzer and started buzzing his hair. She was using a guard so it looked like he was getting a crew cut. I told her, "Honey, take the guard off. You need to remove all his hair. You have to make him bald."

Kenneth also told her, "Yes, Mom, bald."

She reluctantly did as he asked. This was when reality set in for her. She was buzzing her precious son's hair off. After she was done, Kenneth thanked her, and off he went back to his room. After he left, my wife lost it. She cried and cried; she realized that her only son had cancer. I consoled her and told her, "Don't worry. His hair will grow back." She knew that, but the reality of the situation overwhelmed her.

Then I got another letter from the insurance. This time it stated that after November 30, 2015, our insurance was no longer available. On December 1, 2016, they were out of business. Great, we had a contract with the insurance company that was supposed to be in effect until January 1, 2016, but now the contract was breached because it was no longer in business. Nothing I could do. I couldn't sue. How could I? They were bankrupt. Now I had to get insurance.

Thank the good Lord that preexisting condition is no longer a factor; otherwise, I'd be bankrupt. My employer got his broker to look for insurance for us. We were offered several plans. Most of these plans were not accepted by NSHOA. It turns out that they won't accept any of the plans off the marketplace, which was what evidently all these were. You see, my employer is considered a small-group employer, and the insurance companies, in an effort to make Obamacare ineffective, don't offer small businesses any plans. So the plans that were offered weren't any use to me. Then one plan offered to us was a plan called Oscar of New York. They are in partnership with the MagnaCare system. Déjà vu. So was my previous plan. Oscar is another start-up company just like my previous one. Believe it or not, NSHOA accepts this plan, so what choice did I have? I enrolled with them. I prayed to God they didn't go out of business also.

Then we got the bill from the pharmacy that supposedly supplied the chemo drugs to NSHOA for the 177 dollars that was the copayment. This of course was in Kenneth's name, so we reluctantly paid it. Then we got more bills for all the tests that were done and Brookhaven Hospital for his operations; we paid them also. These were the copayments through Health Republic, not the actual cost of the chemo, which was much higher. You see, when he was billed through the facility, the chemo was covered in full. Now that we got the chemo through a pharmacy, we now had to pay a copayment.

Then Kenneth went to his fourth treatment. It went pretty well, no big side effects. His only complaint was being worn out again. Then that same night, Kenneth got nauseous. I gave him both nausea medicines, but he felt no better. I put out a call to his oncologist, who sent a prescription to a pharmacy that was open late. I went to get the medicine. While I was gone, Kenneth had an episode of vomiting, which my wife experienced. She too felt helpless as she could not do anything but try to comfort him. I gave Kenneth his new medication. Finally, he felt better and fell asleep, thank God. He again slept most of the next three days, as the pattern repeated itself. So ended his second cycle. Four more to go, or eight chemo treatments left. God help us.

Kenneth seemed to be going through the same pattern. He tended to sleep for most of the three days after chemo. I think it was partly he felt lousy and partly because it was a mental thing, and the three days went quicker. But I got to tell you, with every dose, he seemed paler. His eyes seemed more sunk in and dark. His nails were getting brittle, and the color was like a grayish color. Poor thing, I knew what he was going through was rough. But he was young and he was strong and he had got a positive attitude. I'm very proud of him.

At this point the oncologist wanted to monitor his lungs closely. So we were now instructed to take him to the pulmonologist in between every chemo treatment. Of course, we did what was recommended. So we took him to the pulmonologist. Kenneth was put through his breathing test that checked the condition of his lungs. Thank God his lungs were still good.

The oncologist wanted Kenneth to have a PET scan done to see if he was responding to the treatment. We of course had to wait for prior approval from the insurance company, which we got after several days. I called the facility where he was to have it done. They had nothing for that week, which was the week of Thanksgiving. He was scheduled for December 1, 2015. I told them that Health Republic was no good as of December first. She said that was okay because he had a prior approval. We had a nice, quiet Thanksgiving. We gave thanks that Kenneth was on his long road to recovery.

On November 27, which was the day after Thanksgiving, he started his third cycle, or his fifth dose. He again got nauseous and had violent vomiting. I again felt helpless. All I could do was comfort him as best as possible. The nurses again tried to control the vomiting and finally were able to control it. So came the end to the treatment. He was again worn out and wanted to go home to sleep.

When we arrived home, I settled Kenneth in, gave him nausea medicine, and told him to make sure he hydrated himself, and he went to sleep. My wife then told me that the radiology center called and wanted to speak with Kenneth. She gave me the name and number of the person that called. I imagined it was to confirm the appointment and to go over his diet the day prior to the procedure.

I called the facility, and to my surprise, I was told that Kenneth's PET scan had to be cancelled because his insurance was expired. She asked me if Kenneth had any other insurance. I said, "Yes, he's an Oscar member, and it goes into effect December first."

"Well, we are going to have to reschedule."

I told her, "When I made the appointment, I told the person that his insurance is no good as of December 1. She told me that this didn't matter because he had a prior approval and it was good until February 2016."

"This is incorrect. As of December 1, the insurance is no longer valid. We have to reschedule, and you have to get a new prior approval."

I told her, "I would no longer use your facility," and I hung up the phone.

I was annoyed. I was now in a situation that I needed to have A PET scan done before December 3. I had to wait till December 1 to get a prior approval with Oscar, his new insurance. There was no way this was going to happen. So I found another facility that took Health Republic. I called the facility, and a very nice woman answered. I told her my situation. She assured me that they could accommodate him. She looked up the schedule and scheduled him for Sunday, November 29. I then told her that the prior approval I had was for another facility. She again reassured me, "Don't worry, we will have the insurance change the location." I asked her if they would do it or if I should do it. "We will take care of everything, don't worry," she said.

"God bless you," I said.

There was a problem, however. Kenneth had his chemo on the twenty-seventh, and he wasn't feeling so great yet. He was upset that he had to get his PET scan so soon after his chemo. He was aware that he was to be given a radioactive isotope that was used to highlight the cancer in his lymph nodes. He was also to be given a dye, and both were to be given intravenously. He felt that he wasn't up to this quite yet. Unfortunately, we had no other choice; he had to have it done. Levia also had concerns; she thought that the infusion he was to get would interfere with the chemo. To this I had no answer, so I put out a call to the doctor. When we got the call back, we were told that it would be no problem, that he could have the PET scan done. So when Sunday came, I took Kenneth to the facility, and he had the PET scan done. Poor kid, feeling terrible as he was, he endured this situation like a champ.

By this time we got his new insurance. We were now members of the Oscar insurance of New York. Thank heaven that Obamacare took the preexisting condition off the table. So Kenneth was now able to get his necessary treatment, and he was covered. This also changed the game again. We no longer had to deal with the copayments. NSHOA was now going to bill the insurance company for his medicine. The only problem was that his anti-nausea medicine was considered a specialty drug. We used to pay a sixty dollars copayment through Health Republic. Now through the Oscar plan, we were required to pay $150, more than double.

The day came for Kenneth to see his oncologist again. We were a bit anxious that day. We were going to get the results of his PET scan. We arrived in the facility and checked in. Soon Kenneth's name was called. They drew his blood, which was what was usually done. Then we went to a room to await the doctor. He came in a while later; he greeted us and sat down. He asked us if we had seen the results of the PET scan. We told him we did not. Then he said that Kenneth was responding quite well to the treatment. I can't tell you how relieved we were to hear that, because there are no words to express that feeling. He said that the report stated that almost all the affected lymph nodes that were affected were normal. The only ones that remained were several that were still swollen around the lungs. We were relieved at the news. Then the doctor asked what Kenneth thought about the good news. Kenneth very nonchalantly said that was kind of what he expected to hear.

Then the doctor told us that Kenneth would be given one more cycle, or two more chemo treatments, and then he was going to order another PET scan. Depending on the results, then decisions had to be made. Do we decide to finish the six cycles? Do we add radiation to the mix? All depends on how the next PET scan results showed. "So let's do the fourth cycle and let's see what happens." He finished his examination, and we went home.

Finally we got good news, and we had a reason to celebrate. So we spent the weekend spreading the good news to the family. Kenneth and I spent the weekend playing Dawn of War video game. This weekend was a happy weekend, the happiest we had since this whole ordeal started. We gave thanks to God that our only son was well on his way to recovery. Hallelujah!

Then back to reality, chemo day came again. Kenneth started his fourth cycle, or his seventh dose of chemo. Unfortunately, it fell on Christmas Eve, so our Christmas was blue. It was again a difficult one. Kenneth again got nauseous and threw up. We went through a difficult ordeal. Again I felt helpless to do anything. I really didn't know how much more of this I could take. Not to mention the suffering that my son was going through. He said to me, "Dad, I can't take much more of this."

I answered, "I hear you, but I'm proud of you. I know that it's not easy, but you are getting better. Try to hang in there. That's why they say battling cancer."

Then he replied, "I am going to beat this damn cancer and go back to living a normal life."

I felt an amazing feeling of pride; Levia and I have raised a strong individual. Well, he finally got through it, but he was extremely worn out, and it showed.

The following three days he did nothing but sleep. We also took our normal place of sleeping on the couch. I was determined that he would not get sick again. I decided after speaking to the nurse and my sister that I would give him his anti-nausea medicine and his prescribed Ativan, a mild tranquilizer that I had at home before we left for his next treatment. This way when we arrived for the next treatment, he already had nausea medicine in him and he would be calm. Slowly he recovered from the treatment, and finally he was back to normal.

The day for his follow-up doctor's visit came. Because of the New Year holiday, it wasn't until January 5, 2016, that the appointment was made. We went again to see the oncologist. His blood was drawn as usual, and we went to the examination room. The doctor came in and examined Kenneth. He reminded us that we needed to have the PET scan done. I told him that we needed a prior authorization in order to have it done. He said that he would put in the authorization, and he did so. So he said, "Let's wait and see, and let's hope for the best." He finished the examination, and we left.

The next day was January 6, 2016. This marked the eleventh anniversary of Manny's death. This was a sad day for us. No matter how many years had gone by, the pain and anguish of his death were still there. We kind of learned to go on with our lives, but we never forgot, and the pain was as strong as ever. We went to the grave and brought flowers that we placed on the grave. Manny's girlfriend before he died also left him flowers. This is something she has done every year since he died. She brings him flowers on his birthday and on his death anniversary without fail. That really means a lot to us, more than words can express.

The morning of January 8, this was Friday, chemo day. This marked the end of his fourth cycle. I gave Kenneth his meds as I decided I would do. This made a remarkable difference in the treatment. He went through his treatment without problems. In fact, it was the easiest time he had ever had going through chemo. He was given his chemo, and he was ready to leave. I stopped at the desk and told the nurse that we had received the authorization for the PET scan the day before. The nurse called the facility for us and made the appointment for him. It was scheduled for January 12 at 12:45 a.m. She gave me a script for the procedure, and she gave one for a pulmonary function test and one for the echo of his heart. So we had a gauntlet of tests to take care of in a span of a week.

Kenneth went for his PET scan, and he also had an echo of the heart done that same day. Unfortunately, there were several hours in between the two procedures. The poor kid was feeling foul because of the aftereffects of the chemo. So he sat for several hours to have both procedures done. Finally, he got them done. We got a copy of them, and we went home. Then we got the pulmonary function test done later in the week. We were done; the gauntlet of tests were over. There was nothing else to do but sit and wait for the report to be done and wait for the results.

Finally we went to see Dr. Syali. We were a bit nervous, then he told us that his results were even better than the last. We let out a sigh of relief. He went on to say that Kenneth was to have two more cycles, or four more chemo infusions. This hit Kenneth like a ton of bricks falling on his head. He thought it was over; now he had to go through four more treatments. We scheduled Kenneth for his remaining chemo appointments, and we went home. Needless to say, Kenneth's demeanor changed; he wasn't happy at all. He was under the impression that he was done with his chemo. So we made the necessary appointments to get him back on the schedule.

Kenneth spent the rest of the day in isolation in his room. He was very angry with the fact that he was going to be getting another two cycles of chemo. He wasn't very pleasant to be around that day. I knew why, though. He had to have more poison, and it was starting to take its toll on him. He was getting exhausted of the whole thing, and I didn't blame him. That's when he finally told me, "Dad, I'm tired of this."

I said, "I know it's been tough, but that's why they say fighting cancer."

"It's easy for you to say. You don't have to go through it," he said.

I wanted to say that I was suffering along with him, but I held back that statement.

Then he told me, "The best way I can explain what I feel is it feels like I'm dead. I have no feeling at all. I feel like a zombie."

"I know it's hard for you, but you are getting cured. Just a bit longer, just two more cycles," I said.

"Just!" he said.

I felt sorry for him. I told him, "Kenneth, if I could, I would trade places with you. I would in a heartbeat." This calmed him down, but he was irritable for the rest of the day.

Then the start of the fifth cycle came, and as was usual, I woke him up. He got ready, and we went to the clinic. He went through his usual four poisons, one right behind the other. With every dose, he was getting paler and paler, almost a gray appearance. His eyes were sunk in, and they got a black appearance, like he had gotten punched in the eyes. He got a bit nauseous, but it wasn't as bad as usual. By the end, the poor kid was so worn out, more so than in the past. The chemo was starting to take its toll on him. After it was over, it was hard for him to walk to the car. Then I got him home, and this time he didn't start feeling better till after the fourth day. The norm was three, so he was physically getting weaker. My wife and I period-ically checked on him constantly.

Then by the second week, he developed a fever. This was the worst-case scenario. This was Thursday, the night before he had to finish his fifth cycle. It was about 10:00 p.m., and I put out a call to Dr. Syali. Then about ten minutes later, our house phone rang. It was the doctor that was on call. I immediately picked up the phone. The doctor identified himself and asked me what had happened. I told him that Kenneth had gotten a fever. I told him his temperate was 100.6, which was just above the threshold of 100.5. He was immediately concerned and told me to hold on while he brought up his chart. He looked up Kenneth's records and noticed that his white blood count was extremely low. He told me something I already knew, and that was his immune system was nonexistent. He asked me if Kenneth was on antibiotics. I told him that he was, that he was put on Cipro and that Kenneth was taking it twice a day without fail. I also told him that I had given him Tylenol to bring the fever down. He told me that was okay and that I acted properly.

He then asked me which emergency room was nearest to where I lived. I told him Brookhaven Hospital. As you know, I can't stand that hospital. My wife really hates that place. That, as you know, is where Manny was ignored. He then instructed me to take Kenneth there as soon as possible. The doctor then told me that he would call the hospital and give them instructions. This way, he will be expected. I thanked him, and he told me, "Don't worry, he'll be fine." I thanked him again. I went to Kenneth's room, and he already knew that he was going to be taken to the hospital. He got ready, as did my wife and I, and we left to the emergency room.

When we arrived, it was about 11:30 p.m. I parked the car, and we went into the ER. No sooner had we entered through to door, the receptionist at the desk asked, "Is this Kenneth?"

Surprised, I said, "Yes, it is."

They immediately took him into the triage area. They took his temperature and his blood pressure. Then he was put in a wheelchair and taken immediately to a private room in the emergency room. Kenneth was placed in isolation.

Kenneth had what is called neutropenia, which basically means that his immune system was nonexistent. The chemo therapy destroyed the white blood cells in his blood. The white blood cells are the natural way a human body fights off infection. Since his white blood cells were extremely low, he couldn't fight off any infection. Then the second thing the body does is cause a fever; it literally tries to burn off the infection. This is called neutropenic fever. His body was literally burning itself up. If this condition wasn't treated, it can be fatal.

Kenneth was put on Cipro, which is a broad-spectrum antibiotic, when he started his chemotherapy. He was taking it religiously every day twice a day. This was prescribed to help him to fight off infection. Kenneth was also placed in isolation by us. He only went to the clinic and back home. We did this because we were warned that he could get sick easily. Kenneth was sick enough with the cancer, and we didn't want him to get any sicker. So we as a family decided to place him under home isolation. It worked out well up to this point, but now that he was at the tail end of his chemo, it was taking its toll on Kenneth's body. I hate to say this, but Kenneth looked like he was a zombie, the living dead. He was thin as rail; he only weighed about 112 pounds. He also, like I said before, had this pale look about him, almost gray in appearance. He also had these hollow eyes that had a black tinge around them. This as a parent was very difficult for me to see. Can you imagine how this affected Levia?

An army of health-care professionals rushed to Kenneth to tend to him. There were x-ray technicians that were already there to take an x-ray of his chest. There was a phlebotomist there to take out blood to run tests. He drew blood to do blood cultures to see what type of infection had developed. He had to draw the blood from Kenneth's arm, which didn't make him happy at all. He kept saying, "I have a port. Draw it from the port." This they could not do because they needed permission from the oncologist on call. Kenneth told them, "Then call him and get permission," which they did, but they didn't get permission in time to get the blood from his port.

The emergency room physician then came to evaluate him. This is when I noticed that everyone that went in to see Kenneth had to gown up, put on latex gloves, and put on face masks. Not for their protection, but for Kenneth's. They didn't want to expose him to anything else. Then a sign was put on his door that stated Isolation. There were also instructions to wash hands before and after entering and leaving. It also stated Mask Required, and gown also was required. Also, believe it or not, no fresh flowers allowed. Kenneth was being attended to in a manner I never expected.

The person from the billing office was there looking for insurance information. This is one thing I can never get used to. How dare this person be there? Let them take care of Kenneth first then worry about insurance. But no, like leaches, the payment brigade is there, ready to draw blood from a stone. I took charge of giving this individual the information required. But in all seriousness, I hold no malice to this person. She was just doing her job. It's the hospital I have the issue with. I got to tell you, anytime I hear anyone ask me what insurance the patient has, my blood boils. It just brings back bad memories of Manny. This is always the first question out of everyone's mouth when you go to any health-care professional's office. That and "You owe $x$ amount of dollars for your copayment, which by the way you have to pay before anything is done." Sound familiar?

Listen, I realize that health care is expensive, and since we are a "for profit system," which I don't agree with, the bill must be paid. I just don't believe that this should be the first thing that comes out of their mouths. That's like if you enter a restaurant, for example, and the first question they ask you is how you will be paying for your food; this just isn't done. Therefore, I believe that the patient should at least be stabilized or evaluated first before this question is asked. It kind of makes you wonder if this decides what kind of care you are going to get. Shame on them! Why don't they come up with a better way to handle this? By the way, part of the reason health care is so expensive is because we are a "for profit system." We'll get into that aspect a little later.

Anyway, the emergency room physician came in and evaluated Kenneth. By this time, they had already gotten permission to use Kenneth's port. The nurse started an intravenous line and hung an

IV bag. The doctor ordered two different antibiotics that were to be given intravenously. These were both broad-spectrum antibiotics and, between the two, would cover just about every infection under the sun. The doctor came to talk to us. She told us Kenneth was neutropenic and that he was to be admitted to the hospital until his fever and infection were brought under control. She asked us if we had any questions; we didn't, then she left.

We then let the nurses know that Levia and I were Kenneth's health-care proxy. We asked to fill out the necessary papers. The papers were given to us, which we filled out and signed. Kenneth was also required to sign them. The signatures were witnessed, and the witnesses signed them also. We were given a copy to show that we were officially his health-care proxies. So from that moment on, we were the ones who made all the decisions concerning his care, even though we already were. This is what Kenneth wanted, and we honored his decision. He had enough on his plate, and he didn't want to deal with anything else.

We waited around until he got a room. He as well as we were quite exhausted. Around 2:30 a.m., the hospital transporters came to get him and take him to a room. We went up with him to get him settled. When we arrived, he was put into his bed. The nurse's aide and the nurse came in and introduced themselves. They started taking his vitals, which by this point Kenneth was totally exhausted. When he was finally settled, we let him get some sleep, and we left. It was now after 3:00 a.m. When my wife and I got home, we both felt that a part of us was missing. I know, I didn't sleep much that night. I was tossing and turning. Finally, out of sheer exhaustion, I fell asleep. Maybe a better way to say this is, I passed out.

The next day we were startled out of bed when the phone rang; it was Kenneth. He wanted to give us an update about his care. We asked him if he slept well. He said that he didn't. He complained about that every time he was falling asleep, he was awakened by someone to take medicine or take more blood or hang another antibiotic. It doesn't seize to amaze me how you never get rest at a hospital. We asked if there was anything special he wanted us to bring him. He wanted his laptop and extra socks because his feet were cold.

We told him we would see him later, and he hung up. I looked at the clock; it was 8:00 a.m., and I was tired. I didn't sleep much. We got up, and Levia made coffee, which we desperately needed. We ate a light breakfast, and we gathered what Kenneth requested, and we left the house.

When we arrived at the hospital, Kenneth was in his bed. He told us that several doctors had come to see us. One of the doctors was an infectious control doctor. Also one of the doctors from his oncology group came. The third was our family doctor. Kenneth's fever was down, but he was still on IV antibiotics. We asked Kenneth if the doctors told him anything. He then told us that they were just routine questions. He also said that the oncologist was going to give him a shot to boost his immune system. Kenneth's statements were very vague, so we decided to put out a call to the doctor. We went to the nurse's station to have the doctor call us as soon as he was able. We were concerned about what exactly was going to be done to Kenneth.

A short time later, the doctor came into his room. As it turned out, he was still in the hospital, making his rounds. We asked him what was going to be done to Kenneth. He explained to us that Kenneth's immune was almost nonexistent. Then he stated that he put in an order to give Kenneth a shot of Leukine that would induce his bone marrow to produce white blood cells. This way he could fight off infection on his own. We asked him if there was any side effects. "Mainly bone pain, but also nausea, dizziness," he said. Then we asked him why it wasn't used during his chemotherapy. He told us, "One of his chemo drugs, bleomycin, causes lung toxicity. Since he was doing well up to this point with his Cipro regimen, we don't normally use the Leukine because it makes the toxicity worse."

We asked him, "Then why use it now?"

He said, "Since now he is neutropenic, the benefits outweigh the risks. I saw his last lung function test, and his lungs were in good condition. Therefore I believe the best course of action is to give him the shot and raise his immune system."

We reluctantly agreed to him getting the shot. Kenneth was given the shot a short time later.

The next day, Kenneth's white blood cell count went way up. Since it was Sunday, the nurse told us that he would probably be released by tomorrow, Monday. Kenneth was excited that he was to be released by Monday, but he was already tired of being in the hospital. I couldn't blame him. By chance, later in the afternoon, our family doctor came in; it was quite unexpected. He told us that his white blood cells were in the normal range. This was the first time since he started his chemo that they were normal. Kenneth said, "Well, I want to go home."

Then Dr. Tomasso said, "I quite agree. There are more germs here in the hospital than at home. I will make some calls to see if I can get all the physicians on the same page, and if we all agree, I will send you home."

Kenneth, needless to say, was ecstatic at the news. Then the doctor returned and said, "I wrote your discharge order. You will be going home today." Kenneth was discharged; he spent three days at the hospital.

The following day, Monday, we called Dr. Syali's office. We wanted to get him back on his chemo schedule. We wanted to end the fifth cycle. We were told to bring him in immediately that same day. So we got ready, and off we went to the doctor's office. We met with Dr. Syali, and we discussed his chemo schedule. He was ready to give him his treatment right away.

Kenneth told him, "I'm just getting better. I'm not quite ready to get chemo."

Dr. Syali took pity on him, and he was scheduled for Friday morning. Kenneth was relieved, and his face showed it. We scheduled his appointments, and we went home.

Friday morning came, and this was to be the end of his fifth cycle. Kenneth got up and got ready. He was actually looking well. The extra week of no chemo made a difference in his appearance. I gave him his anti-nausea medicine, and off we went. We went to the infusion area, and he immediately got weighed. He had gained some weight. Yeah! They took his temperature and blood pressure; all was normal. His white blood count was way up, but that wouldn't last long. He got his four doses of chemo, and wham! He got nauseous, and he threw up. We got through it though, and his nausea ended. Thank God! He was hydrated, and his port was flushed. Then we went home.

He immediately went to bed; he was again looking gray. This was getting worse for us to see. This was also taking its toll on me. I can only imagine how Kenneth was holding up. Judging by his physical appearance, he wasn't doing well. He slept the better part of three days, which, as you know, was his normal routine. He only woke up for hydration, taking his meds, and going to the bathroom. Then he would slowly start to recover. It seems, however, that he was taking a little longer with each dose. This time, by Wednesday, he was feeling better. He was really battling cancer, and he was getting weary. We still had two more treatments to go. It sounded easy, but it wasn't.

Friday came, and it was time for his checkup at Dr. Syali's office. Kenneth got up and said, "Great, the vampires are going to draw blood that I need again." We got ready and went to the clinic. When we went to the infusion area, Kenneth was weighed, and his blood pressure and temperature were taken. Then his blood was drawn, just as he expected. We then went to the examination room. Dr. Syali entered and told us the usual news. Kenneth's white blood count was in the toilet again. There was no surprise there. He told Kenneth to start his antibiotics again. He examined Kenneth physically. Then he told us, "See you guys next Friday, to start his sixth and final cycle." Two more treatments, I thought, and no more poison.

We spent the week as we always did. I worked Monday through Thursday in the morning. We spent our time together playing Dawn of War on our computers. We set up a LAN so we could play together, and we forgot about cancer and chemo for the time being. Kenneth was starting to feel better day by day. He was starting to get his color back; that gray color was finally going away. Those horrible sunken black eyes also started going away. He was starting to look my son, except he was still bald. Then before we knew it, that dreadful day was upon us. Friday was our favorite day of the week. You know, the saying "Thank God it's Friday." But now with chemo being given on Fridays, it kind of put a dampener on it.

Well, it finally arrived, Friday morning and chemo day. It did, however, mark the start of sixth and final cycle. We were nearly at the end. I woke up Kenneth, and he got up; he was a bit grumpy. I can't say I blame him. Kenneth and I got ready to go; I wasn't looking forward to seeing him get sick and looking like the walking dead, especially since he was looking so much better. I know he wasn't looking forward to get his treatment, but he got dressed and got ready to face the music like a man. I got to tell you, I am so proud of him. I can't imagine what I would do in his place. I gave Kenneth his anti-nausea medicine. Levia got his necessity bag ready, his ice chips and drinks, and the baked goods for the staff. Kenneth got his iPod ready, and I did the same and we left.

When we arrived, we went to the back, and we found an area that two recliners were available. They immediately took his vitals as usual and drew blood. The nurse came and started his IV line to his port. When his blood results arrived, the doctor looked them over and approved his chemo treatment. The nurse gave him his premeds, and so it started. She gave him his chemo one by one. Kenneth was getting paler and paler, and he got sick again. We all tended to him as necessary, and we got the nausea under control. With every dose, I was watching my only son turn into a zombie again. He again was sickly gray in appearance and had hollow eyes. I stayed strong even though I was dying inside.

I aged another ten years through this whole experience. He was finally done. He was hydrated, and off we went home. I had to help Kenneth into the Suburban. This was the first time that I had to do this. Poor kid, with every treatment, he got weaker than the time before. I got him home and helped into his bed, and right to sleep he went. I woke him only to give him his meds as needed. Thank God he had only one treatment left. If we could only get through the next two weeks without getting a fever, it would be great.

One week went by and we went to see Dr. Syali for his regular post-chemo checkup. The usual was done—blood work, blood pressure, etc. This time when they took his temperature, he had a slight fever. This concerned Dr. Syali, but the temperature wasn't at the point to get hysterical over. I was told to monitor his temperature often, and hopefully it wouldn't get any higher. He wanted us to get another pulmonary function test done, and he gave us the order for it. He told us that if all stayed well, he would be getting his last dose of chemo done the following Friday, and we left. Finally, I thought, his last dose of chemo.

When we arrived home, I immediately schedule his pulmonary function test, which was set for Thursday, the day before chemo. The tech that did the test was gracious, and she worked around Kenneth's schedule. He was treated like a king there. She came in special just for Kenneth. I monitored his temperature every couple of hours. I did it so often it was driving Kenneth crazy. Saturday went by, and his temperature stayed just below the threshold of 100.5 degrees Fahrenheit. By Sunday morning, however, my worst fears came true. I took Kenneth's temperature, and it reached 101.6 degrees Fahrenheit. I took him to the NSHOA facility in Setauket, which was the only one that was open on Sunday.

We were told by Dr. Syali when we saw him on Friday to bring him into the facility, telling us that we could do here whatever the hospital did. Well, to our surprise, when they saw him, he had such a high temperature' it was 101.6 and holding. We were immediately instructed to take him to the hospital. I was extremely annoyed, and Kenneth was furious. "I was told to bring him to NSHOA by Dr. Syali, saying that you guys can do whatever the hospital does here." They said he needed IV antibiotics immediately.

I took him to Brookhaven Hospital as instructed. We knew the routine by this point. The weather was getting lousy a blizzard was coming to Long Island. It was to start Sunday night into Monday, and it was to be a big one. Anyway, we arrived at the emergency room, and they took him right in. He again was isolated, and all the tests were done again. Kenneth had neutropenic fever again. He was admitted, and it started all over again. This time, however, he was to stay a week. We stayed with him the entire day, and later in the evening, he finally got a room. This time he got a room with only one bed in it. The last time he had a room with two beds, but he was the only one in the room. This room was really nice. It was, as we found out later, reserved for women that have breast cancer. We settled him in and left; it was about 9:30 p.m. When we left, the snow had started, but it wasn't bad yet.

The next day he called us early. He wanted us to bring his laptop and some snacks from home. The blizzard had arrived, and there were several inches of snow on the ground. I promised him that I would get to him. Luckily, I have a full-size Suburban with four-wheel drive. Levia got his things ready while I cleaned the snow off the truck. A short time later, we set off to the hospital. The roads were covered with snow, but the truck plowed through the snow with no effort. I took my time of course, and we finally arrived. Levia went upstairs and gave him his things. I decided not to go up, mainly because of the blizzard. The snow was coming down very heavy, and visibility was bad. Levia told him that we weren't going to stay because of the snow. She came down about fifteen minutes later, and we returned home, trekking through the snow carefully.

I wasn't happy that we weren't able to see Kenneth that day. The blizzard had dumped about sixteen inches of snow. When the snow had finally stopped, I had the pleasure of cleaning up the walkways and driveway. Thankfully, I have a snow blower, and it did make the job easier. It still took a while. I helped several neighbors clear out the entrances of their driveways. The snowplows had really dumped a lot of snow in this area, and digging with shovels really took effort. So I did the neighborly thing and helped as much as I could. Levia and I spent the day at home in constant contact with Kenneth.

The next day was Tuesday, and we went to the hospital. Kenneth lit up like a Christmas tree. He was so happy we were visiting him. He was looking better, but he was still running a fever. It wasn't as high as it was when he was admitted. He complained about the hospital food; he didn't care for it much. He also complained about being bored, so I called and got his TV connected. We asked us if he was seen by any of the doctors. He said that Dr. Tomasso was the only one so far that had come to see him. So we settled in, and we kept him company.

A short time later, Dr. Syali came into the room and examined Kenneth. Kenneth was angry at him and said, "I thought you guys were able to treat me at the clinic."

He apologized to Kenneth, telling him that once the fever started, he needed IV antibiotics around the clock. He told us that he wasn't going to give Kenneth the shot he got the last time to boost his immune system. He was concerned about the lung toxicity; we were going to have to wait until his white blood cells went up on their own accord. Then he told us that he probably had to stay for the rest of the week. He wasn't going to be released until he was no longer neutropenic. This of course did not make Kenneth happy. Dr. Syali finished his checkup and left. Kenneth was really sad of the fact that he was going to stay for a week in the hospital. Then I remembered his pulmonary function test on Thursday. Since the tech came in on her day off to do this for Kenneth, I cancelled the appointment. I didn't want her to make a trip when Kenneth was still in the hospital.

We spent the entire day with Kenneth, watching TV and talking. We tried our best to make his stay as pleasant as possible. We only left his side when we ate lunch and dinner. Then a short time later, a nurse's aide came in and told us that Kenneth was going to be transferred to another room. My wife asked her why this was being done; we were settled in already. She said that this room was being given to a patient that had breast cancer. My wife, like a lioness, immediately said, "Kenneth has cancer also. I don't want him moved." The aide said a nurse would come in shortly and explain the situation. When the nurse entered the room and my wife again said, "I don't want my son moved," the nurse didn't argue much and left.

Then the head nurse came in with the same story about the room being given to a breast cancer patient. Then my wife said, "My heart goes out to the person that has breast cancer, but Kenneth has cancer also. He is comfortable right here. I don't want him moved. Besides," she said, "he is supposed to be in isolation, and this is a private room. This is the best room for him." Then my wife told the nurse of our experience with this hospital and how they didn't take care of Manny because he had no health insurance. She also said how we detested the hospital and how this was fueling that feeling. Finally, after some fanfare, it was decided that Kenneth was not to be moved. My wife definitely is a force to be reckoned with. We spent the rest of the day at the hospital with Kenneth.

Kenneth did spend the rest of the week in the hospital. We kept him company every day from morning to evening. We were now getting food for Kenneth to eat. He just didn't care for the hospital food at all and wouldn't eat much of it. I got to tell you, the food choices were deplorable. The end for us was when they gave him a portabella mushroom, a fungus. I wouldn't eat that. I think it's disgusting, yuck! I also don't think that is appropriate for a person that was neutropenic, but that's just my opinion. We were concerned that he would lose more weight, which really wasn't an option; he was skinny as a rail already. We just wanted Kenneth as comfortable as possible. He was battling cancer, which is truly that, a battle. His battle was grueling and taking his toll on him. He is our son, and I was going to do everything in my power to make him comfortable. It's as simple as that!

Finally, the day came for Kenneth to be released from the hospital. He was happy that he was finally leaving this place. Before he was discharged, a nursing supervisor came in and tried to explain why they wanted to move Kenneth. He we were again, and I thought to myself, "Here we go." My wife laced into this woman and went into detail about what had happened to Manny and how we hated this hospital. This clearly blindsided the supervisor, and she went on the defensive. She kept trying to say that this room was reserved for breast cancer patients exclusively. My wife said again, "My son has cancer also. What's the difference? My heart goes out to this poor woman that has cancer. I just don't see the difference. Cancer is cancer," she said.

The supervisor tried in vain to justify the reasoning, but when she realized that she was barking up the wrong tree, she just gave up. Like I said before, my wife is a force to be reckoned with. Don't mess with her. Besides, I agree with her wholeheartedly.

We had to go through the process of getting discharged. It isn't as easy as you may think. It is not as simple as you are being "discharged," here are your "discharge instructions" and then you are sent home. We had to wait to get his IV taken out of his port. Then we had to wait for Dr. Tomasso to write his discharge orders, which he did immediately. Then the nurse had to write up her discharge instructions that took a while. Then probably the longest wait of all was to wait for someone from social service to see if we agreed with Kenneth being discharged from hospital or if we felt they were discharging him prematurely. Finally the person came, and we told him that we agreed with the discharge. We signed some papers, and we finally discharged. The process took about three hours. Too long for Kenneth's liking.

I called Dr. Syali's office to inquire about his chemo schedule. I was told to bring him in on Friday on his regular day, and it would then be decided what was to be done. Friday morning we got up, and we went in for our usual 10:00 a.m. appointment. They drew blood, and the usual pretreatment stuff was done. This time, however, we were taken to the examination room to wait for Dr. Syali. A short time later, he came in, and we discussed the options. He told us that we hadn't gotten the pulmonary function done. He knew that he was to have it done the Thursday when he was at Brookhaven.

Then he said, "We can cancel today's treatment, and you can have the pulmonary test done and then have the chemo next Friday. The other option is to have the chemo done today and omit the bleomycin and give you the other three chemos." He said, "I don't have a problem with that."

I didn't either, because I had discussed the matter with my sister, and in her discussion with her team in North Carolina, they said it was okay to omit the bleomycin, that it wouldn't make a difference in the outcome. Ultimately, though, it was Kenneth's decision to make. Kenneth very clearly stated, "Give me my treatment today. Omit the bleomycin. I don't want to delay this any longer. I decided this morning that no matter what, I was having this done today regardless."

I was so proud of him; he was strong willed, and he just wanted this junk to end. Dr. Syali smiled and said, "Okay, then let's go to the treatment area and get this over with."

Kenneth went to the infusion room and sat in the recliner. He was given his premeds, and the nurse started his chemo. There was a nurse that I had never seen before. She took care of Kenneth; unfortunately, I didn't get her name. When she started giving Kenneth his chemo, she asked him if he had Hodgkin's lymphoma. He answered her yes. Then she said, "Ah, don't worry about it." Kenneth gave her a strange look. Then she told him, "Want me to tell you a secret?" Kenneth said okay.

"I had what you have, and now I'm cured. Don't worry, you are going to be fine."

This seemed to raise Kenneth's spirits higher. He didn't get nauseous this time. He did get gray though, and his eyes got hollow again. He seemed determined not to get sick. I think in his mind he said—and pardon the words, but I know my son—"Fuck you, cancer. I win." He was finally done with his chemo.

For Kenneth it was a long grueling battle, but like the warrior he is, he fought the fight, and he prevailed. He too, like Manny, is my hero. Levia and I had taught them to be of good characters and strong will, and they truly are. Kenneth, I am so proud of you, and I love you. I know I was your chemo buddy, but you ultimately were the warrior. I was just your support. I know your brother would have been proud of you also. God bless you always!

I took Kenneth home, and to my surprise, he didn't go right to sleep, as was his usual thing. He got on his computer and told all his friends that his chemo was finally over. We too spread the news to everyone. Kenneth was in good spirits. He did look like he had battle fatigue physically, but in his mind, he was strong. I guess it was mind over matter. He didn't sleep until later in the evening. He recovered rather quickly, and his appetite was coming back. His energy was coming back, and by Monday, he was his usual self again. The only lingering question was, did he need radiation treatment also? That thought kind of lingered in my mind. I'm sure it was on Kenneth's mind also, but we didn't talk about it. We were relishing the accomplishment he had made.

Friday rolled along again, and it was time to see Dr. Syali again. We went through the usual routine, and we went to the examination room, awaiting Dr. Syali. He came in a short time later, and the first thing he did was smile at Kenneth. "Congratulations, Kenneth, your chemotherapy is over. I know I put you through a lot and asked much of you and your parents," he said. "But you went through it like a champ, and you had a great support team." He was referring to

Levia and me. "We will miss your mother's baking, but I am glad to see you strong and well on your way recovery."

My wife baked for the crew on chemo day and sent them baked goods every chemo day without fail. This was our way of saying thanks for their dedication. He also gave us an order to have a PET scan again. "We will let you know when the approval from Oscar comes in."

Now he said, "I will refer you to a radiation oncologist and see if you need radiation treatment." I asked him if he thought he would need it. He said, "He might. Remember, Kenneth was really sick when he came in, but he responded to the chemo well. Let's wait and see. He gave us a referral to see Dr. Joseph Cirrone. He told us that he was in the other side of the facility. I went back there and made an appointment for Kenneth. We were told to bring in his last PET scan.

When the day came to see Dr. Cirrone, we went with anticipation to see him. We went into the examination room. Dr. Cirrone came in and introduced himself. He was a very nice man. He examined Kenneth and then asked us if we had the PET scan. I handed all the PET, scans not just the last. Then he looked at Kenneth's entire records. He was very thorough; he looked at everything. Then he looked at all the PET scans. When he saw the first one, he said, "Wow." The scan showed how bad the cancer was. His entire chest area was lit up like a Christmas tree. He showed us the scan and explained everything, showing us what was what. "All these areas of light are the lymph nodes that are cancerous." He read the report and said, "Wow, the largest swollen lymph node was 8 cm. That's large." He looked at the PET scan again and said, "I don't see it here."

He then asked us, "Was a biopsy done?"

We told him, "Yes, it was done early on."

He looked in his records again and found the pathology report and read it. "Ah, good, they removed this one when they did the biopsy. So that's not part of the equation, and that's good," he said. He then looked at the second PET scan. This was the one taken to see if the chemo was working. He looked it over and said, "The chemo treatment was working well." He then showed us and explained everything as he showed us the scan. There was a huge difference in the glowing areas; they were all almost gone. He looked at the report, and he was happy with the results. Then he looked at the third scan and report. These were the latest ones we had. It was taken right after his fourth cycle was completed. He looked it over and said, "He's clean. There is nothing left." He showed us and explained what we were looking at as he went along.

Then he asked us, "He had six cycles done, correct?" We answered yes. Then he said, "That's four more treatments. Well," he said, "I'm leaning toward not treating him with radiation. I can't imagine that with four more treatments to see anything. Especially since this one shows clean." Then he explained what was to be done if radiation was done. He explained the risks involved and said it was to be done once a week at the same time for four weeks. He then asked us, "When is his next PET scan scheduled for?" We told him we were waiting for the green light from Dr. Syali and the insurance company. "So let's do this after he gets the PET scan done. Call the office, and we will look it over then. But at this point, I don't feel it's necessary. In the interim I will consult with my colleagues."

We got a card from the receptionist, and she gave us the direct number and we left. Needless to say, we were happy with the news so far.

Then the call we were waiting for finally came in. The approval for his next PET scan had arrived, and we were given an authorization number. I called for an appointment, and it was set for April 16, 2016. When the day arrived, we went to the facility, and Kenneth had his PET scan done. They took him in, and finally it was done. We waited for the copy of the scan, and off we went. We saw Dr. Syali on April 22, and he told us his CAT scan was clean and to make an appointment to see Dr. Cirrone. I did just that, and we were to see him on May 2, 2016.

We went to see Dr. Cirrone and went to the examination room. He came in and examined Kenneth again. Then he looked at the new PET scan, and as expected, he was clean. Then Dr. Cirrone told us that he discussed Kenneth's case with several colleagues, and it was agreed that Kenneth did not need radiation done. He spent his time trying to justify Kenneth getting radiation, but he couldn't find any. Then he looked over to Kenneth and said, "I can give you radiation if you want, even if I can't find a reason to give it."

Kenneth answered, "No, I'm good." Then we thanked the doctor and left. Hurray! Kenneth did not need radiation; we were ecstatic. Levia and I said, "Thank you, God."

Then on May 31, 2016, we went to see Dr. Syali. We went through the usual and went to the examination room to wait for the doctor. When he came in, he greeted us and he told us that he got the news from Dr. Cirrone. He told us, "Kenneth does not need radiation, congratulations." Then he examined Kenneth and told us that his blood looked good. He told Kenneth to stop taking his anti-biotics. Kenneth smiled; he hated taking them anyway. Then he said, "I don't need to see you until three months."

Then I asked the doctor, "Dr. Syali, is Kenneth in remission?"

The doctor answered, "Yes, Kenneth is in remission, congratulations."

We thanked him, and we thanked the entire staff in the infusion room as well as the front office. "Kenneth is in remission," we told everyone, and they were all happy for us. There were tears of joy and lots of hugs and kisses. Kenneth didn't need to see the doctor until September 2016, then another PET scan would be done, and if it came back clean, which my faith in God said yes, he would have his port removed and he would be considered cured. But in the meantime, Kenneth was cancer-free! Thank you, God!

When we left, Kenneth was walking in the clouds. I hadn't seen him smile like that in a long time. My wife and I, as you can imagine, were also right there with him. Then I said, "Hey, Kenneth, this is reason to celebrate. Where would like to go?"

To my surprise, he said, "Take me to Friendly's." I thought he would want to somewhere else, but that was his choice. We all went to Friendly's, and we ate. And funny, we toasted to his good health over ice cream.

Levia and I finally got a good night's sleep that night. We hadn't slept well since this whole ordeal started. Every time Kenneth had his chemotherapy, we would sleep on the couch. This way we would be near him. Our room was on the second floor; his room was on the first floor. We slept in the living room, and if Kenneth needed anything or if he felt sick, he would knock on his wall, and we would run to his side. When he got sick, the fact that he had cancer just was on our minds and we just couldn't sleep, so after nine months since this started, we could finally sleep. What a relief.

Kenneth had it rough since his brother died. He went into a depression soon after his brother's death, and we didn't know how to get him out of it. Levia told me one day that she dreamed of Manny and he told her to get Kenneth a cat. We went to get bird food one day soon after the dream, and in the store, there was a gentleman giving away kittens for adoption. When we looked over the kittens, she immediately came over to us. Needless to say, that's the one we took home. She was a beautiful short-haired red cat with white stripes.

Then we took her home. We placed her down on the floor. She walked over to a shelf where my wife had some pottery. She screeched, and with her front paw, she knocked the piece off the shelf, and it shattered. That was the only thing that she ever broke. Then she went into Kenneth's room like she knew that's where she was supposed to go. We woke up Kenneth and said, "Good morning, Kenneth, look what we brought you." I picked up the cat and placed it on the bed. He smiled from ear to ear. He named her Eres. They were friends from day 1, and she never left his side or his room. He was sent to him from above.

Then ironically several months before he got sick, she got sick, and she stopped eating. I knew that this wasn't a good thing. We took her to the vet, and he thought she had gotten a fur ball stuck in her throat. He gave her some medicine for this, and we took her home. She ate a little for several days, but then she stopped eating again. We took her back to the vet. This time she was jaundice, and he broke the bad news. "She's dying," he said. The decision had to be made: try to revive her (but he didn't recommend that) or put her to sleep. This was Kenneth's cat, so it was his choice. He said, "I don't want her to suffer. Let's put her down." I had to leave the room because the animal lover I am, I can't see that. My wife told me that just before she was put down, she gently touched his cheek while looking directly into his eyes. This was her saying good-bye to him. He lost it and he left. Then she was gently put to sleep.

Now I'm not much of a cat person. I prefer dogs, but she was the nicest cat I have ever had in my household. She was no trouble at all. She was a pleasure to own, and she was Kenneth's best friend. I do believe that she died in Kenneth's place. She graciously gave her life to save Kenneth. I truly believe this, because not to long after this, Kenneth was diagnosed with cancer.

So as you can see, Hodgkin's disease is not as fatal as Manny's doctors and their attorneys tried, at one point, to use as part of their defense. The fact is that Hodgkin's lymphoma is one of the most curable cancers. The odd of being cured from Hodgkin's disease is 80–90 percent. Those are pretty good odds. The fact that they tried to say that Manny would have died from this condition is absurd. Not only that, but he didn't have the disease. I have found out that a person can have genes for certain diseases in their bodies that never manifest themselves. Many stay dormant in the bodies and never become a problem. Of course, we'll never know if Manny would have gotten this disease.

He did have an AVM, and he should have been treated for it. It may not have been curable; not all AVMs are, but at least they could have treated him to reduce the risk of bleeding, which is the risk with any AVM. The bleeding is usually fatal, and thus by reducing the size of the AVMs, it would have reduced the risk of bleeding and possibly stops the seizures. If he would have died by having the embolization done, we could have lived with it. At least they tried. But because of greed, his treatment was delayed and led to his death. That is something we just can't live with. The doctors claim that they were justified in delaying his procedure. Think about this; he was scheduled for his first embolization on November 11, 2004. They cancelled it and didn't reschedule it until February 2005, three months later. Do you seriously believe that it took three months to be able to put Manny on the schedule to treat him? Three months? Doesn't it make more sense that the doctor's figured by February his Medicaid would finally be in place?

Not only that, but the doctors and hospitals knew that charity care was available to treat Manny, and they never said a word about it. They would have gotten paid for his care regardless. This is inexcusable, and they knew this. That is why they settled out of court, because they knew that they would have lost. They tried their best to prevent this, frequently changing their excuses as to why they didn't treat Manny. Our story, however, never changed, because we were telling the truth. You only have to change your story when you are lying, and that's what they were doing, lying. They were like children caught with their hands in the cookie jar and then trying to say they didn't do it.

Here is another disturbing fact; according to Obamacare.com, in a 2012 families USA study, more than 130,000 Americans died between 2005 and 2010, because of their lack of health insurance, the number of deaths due to a lack of coverage averaged three per hour and that the issue plagued every state. Other studies have shown those statistics to be high or low, but all studies agree: In America, the uninsured are more likely to die than those with insurance. Okay, so you are saying, yeah, that's according to ObamacareFacts.com. They skewed the results. Okay, let's look at another study from a private institution.

According to the *Harvard Gazette* (http://news.harvard.edu/gazette/story/2009/09/new-study-finds-45000-deaths-annually-linked-to-lack-of-health-coverage/), nearly 45,000 deaths yearly are associated with the lack of health insurance. Do the math. In the same five-year period as the previous study, the result is, 225,000 Americans died. This is more than the total American soldiers that died during the Vietnam War of 58,209, and during the Korean War, the total number of American soldiers that died was 36,516. The total amount combined between the two wars is 94,725, which is less than the number of Americans that have died in just a five-year period because of lack of health insurance. At least the soldiers were fighting for our freedom. What was the uninsured fighting for? Their lives, that's what! Does this sound right, that this happens here in this country? I sure don't think so. We are the richest country in the world. This should not happen here. Are we at war in this country, a war against our health?

Now the politicians in Washington want us to believe that health care in this country is a privilege and not a right. I guess we can all agree that the politicians are supposed to uphold the Constitution of the United States. In fact, they swear an oath that they will before they take office. So let's read the preamble of our Constitution:

> We, the people of the United States, in order to form a more perfect union, establish justice, insure domestic tranquility, provide for the common defense, promote the general welfare, and secure the blessings of liberty to ourselves and our posterity, do ordain and establish this Constitution for the United States of America.

First, let's look at the word *preamble*. The definition of *preamble* is "a preliminary or preparatory statement; an introduction, stating its purpose, aims, and justification." So we can fairly say it is stating the purpose or aim of our Constitution. Now let's look at the word *promote*. The definition of *promote* is "to further the progress of (something, especially a cause, venture, or aim); support or actively encourage." Now let's look at some synonyms of this word: *encourage, advocate, further, advance, assist, aid, help, contribute to, foster, nurture, develop, boost, stimulate, forward, work for.* Now the word *welfare.* The definition of this word is "the health, happiness, and fortunes of a person or group." Now let's look at synonyms of this word: *well-being, health, comfort, security, protection, prosperity, success, fortune.*

So let's inserts the synonyms into the preamble.

> We, the people of the United States, in order to form a more perfect union, establish justice, insure domestic tranquility, provide for the common defense, promote [encourage, advocate, further, advance, assist, aid, help, contribute to,

foster, nurture, develop, boost, stimulate, forward, work for] the general welfare [well-being, health, comfort, security, protection, prosperity, success, fortune], and secure the blessings of liberty to ourselves and our posterity, do ordain and establish this Constitution for the United States of America.

Are you starting to get the picture? So can we safely say this is what our founding fathers had in mind? Not what our current politicians have molded it into to justify their actions? Besides, it's we the people, not we the government or we the politicians, and by the way, they are elected officials, not our leaders. Therefore, I believe that health care is a right and not a privilege.

I'm sure you realize that the politicians have a "Cadillac" (the best) health-care insurance that pays for everything. Not only that, they have this insurance for their entire life. Do we have this same right? No, we don't! They don't suffer the problems that we as citizens with our health care do. What makes them better than us? Everyone in this country should have access to the same quality health care equally, period. No one, whether you are rich or poor, should have to carry the burden of worrying about what type of care we are going to receive. We should all have access to the same care our elected officials get. We are guaranteed equality in this country, and our health-care system should be no different. I believe in equal care for all.

Therefore, I believe that we should have universal health care in this country. I know what you're saying. I don't want the government making the decisions when it comes to my health. I agree. I don't either. I believe that the decisions should be made between the individual and the doctor, period. The government should not have any say in the decisions at all. I do believe that rather than have a third party (a "for profit" insurance company) pay that, we as a nation should be paying for it. Besides, the insurance companies are making the decisions for you now, and the doctors' hands are tied. How many times do the insurance companies deny payment for a procedure or a drug because they simply don't want to pay for it? So the doctor has to go to an alternate drug or treatment. So you may not realize it, but they have made the decision for you, and when it comes to profits, I don't believe this should be part of the equation at all.

You hear about how are health-care costs are going sky-high. Sure, they are, because of all the profits that have to be made first. Do you think that the insurance companies are in the business because they care for you? If this is what you believe, you have been deceived into believing this. United Health Care made 11 billion dollars in profit in 2015. Do you want to see what that looks like? $11,000,000,000. Whew! That's a lot of zeros! That's just one of many private for-profit health-care insurance companies. They are in the business of making money, and that is all that they care about. They couldn't care less about you or me. Imagine if we took them out of the equation. How much less would we spend as a nation for health care? So we have to put an end to this practice. The sooner the better.

Do you believe we have the best health-care system in the world? Take a moment and think about it. It doesn't. According to Forbes.com, we were ranked eleventh in eleven countries compared. We were dead last. The UK was number 1, and they have universal health care. Number 2 was Switzerland; they have universal health care. Number 3 was Sweden; they have universal health care. Number 4 was Australia; they have universal health care. Tied for the fifth position were Germany and the Netherlands; they both have universal health care. Tied for the seventh position were New Zealand and Norway; they both have universal health care. In the ninth position was France; they have universal health care. Tenth was Canada, and guess what? They also have universal health care. In the eleventh slot was the USA; we have a for-profit health-care system. Seems to me that a universal health-care system beats out our for-profit system.

Not only that, we as a nation spend $8,508 on average per person as compared to the UK that spends $3,405 on average. They spend less, and they were number 1. We spend more than double, and we were dead last. Still think that we have the best system as we are led to believe? Hey, don't take my word for it. Look it up yourself. I didn't make these numbers up. Hey, the Internet is a beautiful thing. Use it and see. Google "Mirror on the Wall 2014" or look it up on Forbes.com. Remember that we will all get sick at one time or another, so I hope you don't care about this serious situation. Because it does affect us all!

Okay, you say that's just one study and it was done by the Commonwealth Fund. Who are they? Okay, let's look at the report from the World Health Organization. They had 190 countries in their list, and the USA came in thirty-seventh on that list. Compared to the rest of world, we weren't in the top 10, not even the top 20 or 30. Then our politicians have the audacity to tell us we have the best. Really? There wasn't any study I looked at, and I looked at many that shows that the USA has the best system, and that's sad. I urge all Americans to wake up before we all fall victims to a less-than-best system. Let's demand universal health care for all. It works in many nations around the world, then why can't we make it work here? Are they better or smarter than us?

Now let's get into the pharmaceutical companies. Kenneth was taking an anti-nausea capsule called Akynzeo. The dose is just one capsule. It works amazingly well; it worked wonders for Kenneth. Well, this one capsule is amazingly expensive, and it is not covered under our health-care insurance. That means I have to pay for it, and that cost doesn't go toward my out-of-pocket cost limit on my insurance plan. This capsule at CVS costs $583.66 for one capsule. This costs $572.43 at Walgreens and $583.95 at Rite Aid. What justifies charging this much for one capsule? Greed! The top ten pharmaceutical companies made 89.8 billion dollars (89,000,000,000) in profits. Starting to see the waste of money we spend on health-care system? I think you get the idea. I won't bore you any longer. I just wanted to show you examples of money that we spend on our health system that go into the pockets of others not into the system.

My health insurance costs about $23,000 a year. I have a platinum plan, which is supposed to be the highest tier that we can buy. This has a $2,000 per person and $4,000 per family out-of-pocket limit, and whatever the insurance company doesn't cover in the plan does not get added to this amount. Example, back to the Akynzeo, the cheapest price was $572.43, times 12 doses, for the twelve treatments, that adds up to $6,869. That figure does not get added to my out-of-pocket cost. Then when Kenneth was in the hospital, his infectious control doctor was not covered by the plan. Apparently he wasn't in the network. His bill was $4,000, and that figure did not go toward his out-of-pocket limit either. Starting to see a trend? Who is the one affected? The patient. That's over ten thousand dollars. So much for the out-o-pocket limits, which, by the way, we still had to pay. Now the figure is over $12,000. Those are just a few examples; there are more. I admit it was less than the $42,000 that Manny was billed for, but it is still significant.

So as you can see, even with health insurance, getting sick in the USA can financially ruin you. This can and probably will happen to everyone. Everyone gets sick at one time or another. Either now or later, every one of us will have a family member require critical care. We are not immortal; we don't live forever, and health insurance does *not* cover everything. So we are all at risk to be financially ruined. So why don't we do something about it? Manny is just one story of many that have gone through the system and paid the price of death. Is this what we want as a nation of rational people? I think not! I know that Obamacare is not the answer. Congress designed it to fail. It does have its advantages, like I stated earlier. It does also have disadvantages. One fact remains clear: we cannot stop soaring health-care costs if we remain a "for profit" system. Health care is *not* a commodity; it's not a product. So why do we treat it as such?

Congress wants to repeal Obamacare; they want to return to the way things were. If this were the case, now Kenneth may not be alive today. We cannot allow the preexisting condition to ever come back on the table, for example. We cannot continue to allow insurance companies to dictate what they will or will not pay for. With Obamacare, I was able to have Kenneth on my policy until he's twenty-six. That, I believe, saved his life, because he was insured through my policy. We have to demand Congress and the president to give us universal health care that pays 100 percent of the cost. Not the current third-party payer, for-profit system. It works around the world. Why not here? We can't survive with the current system; it is inefficient, and it doesn't work. Like I said before, only doctors and patients should make decisions about health-care treatment, no one else. Especially not the government or insurance companies.

I'm not against doctors getting compensated for their expertise. Far from it, I believe they should be well compensated. I do believe, however, that if a person becomes a doctor just to make himself rich, then he/she is going into that profession for the wrong reasons. Physicians and all health-care professionals for that matter are a well-respected profession, and rightly so. They are among the noblest professionals on earth. I myself hold them in high regard, and I respect their honor and integrity. I believe that they were sent here by God to take care of his people. That of course is not only my belief but my opinion as well. Hey, we are all entitled to our opinion.

If we have universal health care in the USA, this would ensure that every single citizen has equal access to health care, the same health care for all; an individual's social status does not matter. This will ensure that no one is financially ruined. Don't let politicians fool you about this matter. I'm sure they are going to bring up the cost issue, and that is a fair point. But you know what? We pay them to take care of this country. It is time they start earning their money and make it work. If we can send billions of dollars to foreign aid to other countries, then we can find the money to make it work. They have to ignore the powerful lobbyist that will no doubt come into play. But they have to remember this it's "We the people," not "We the corporations." And no matter what the Supreme Court says, corporations are *not* people; they are an entity, a for-profit business. That's why we have corporate laws. My fellow Americans, *wake up*, and let's demand change. Let's stop this madness. Thanks for reading.

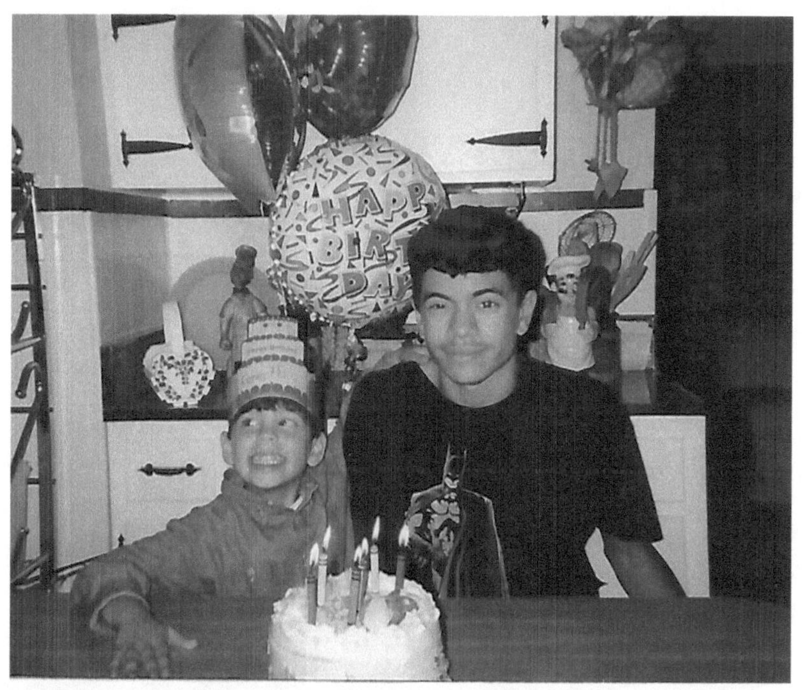

Happy Birthday Kenneth

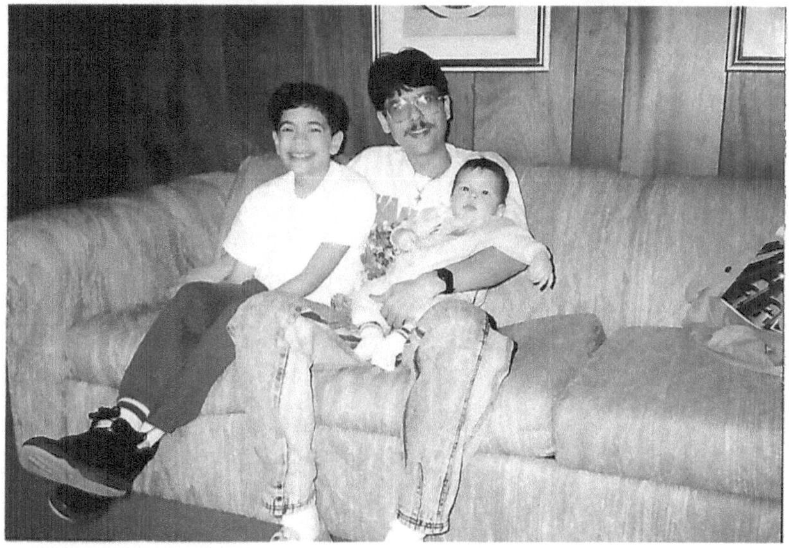

My Two Sons and Me

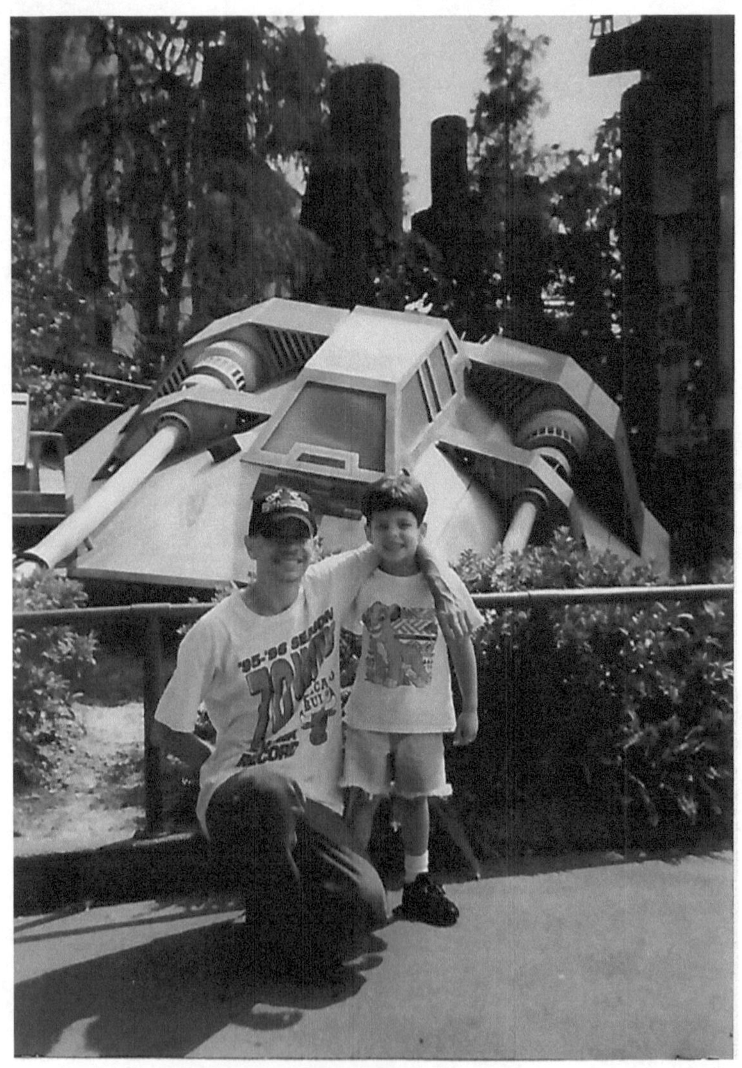

The brothers in Florida

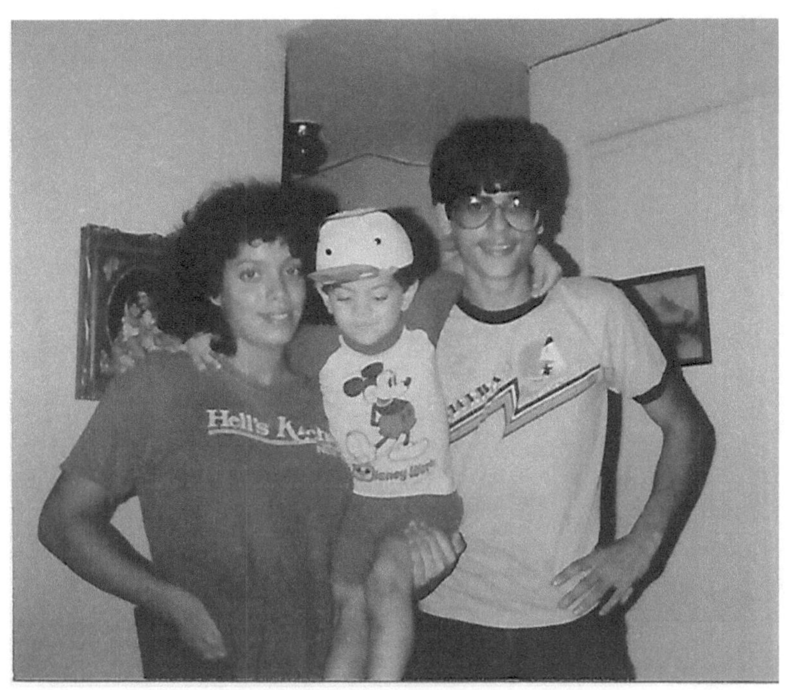

The Family young

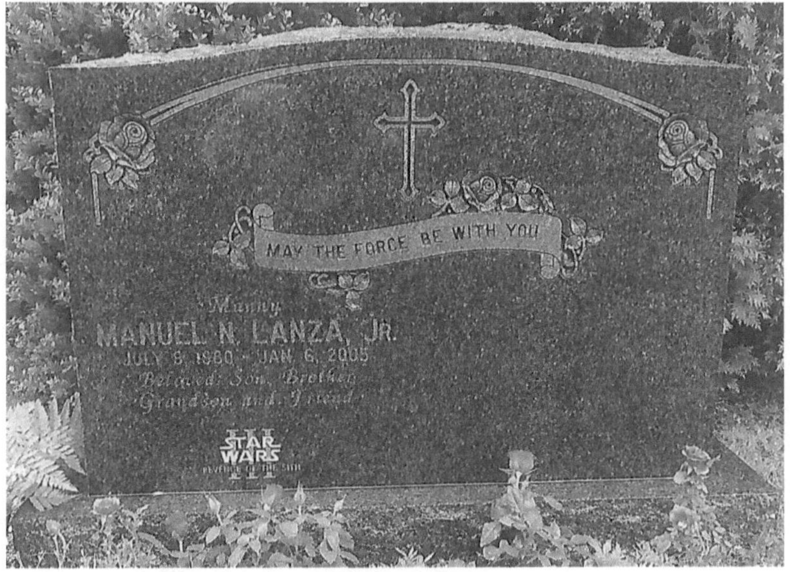


Manny's grave

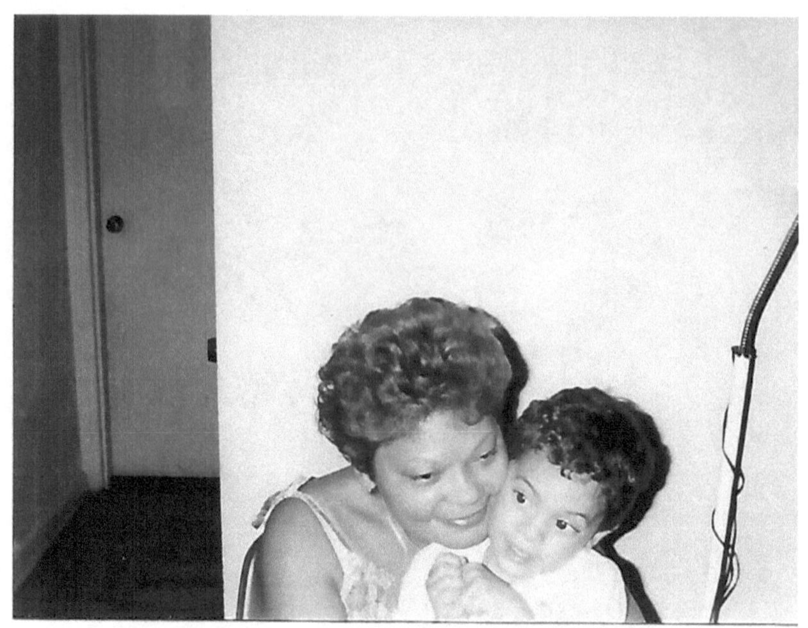

Manny with his paternal grandma

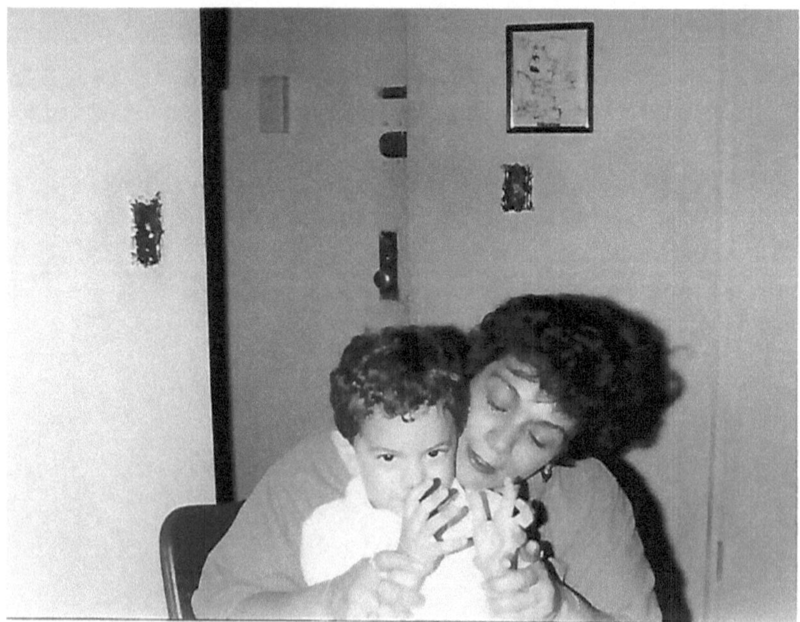

Manny with his maternal grandma

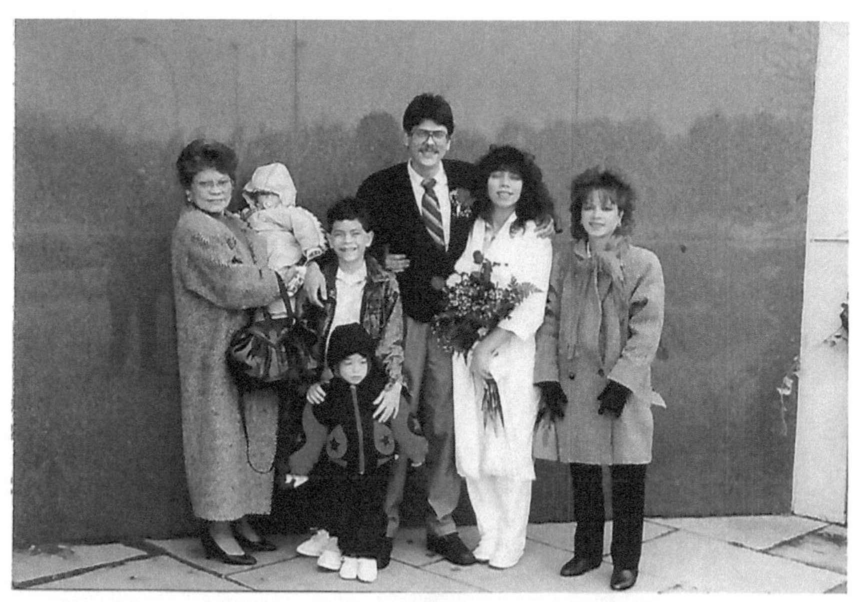

Celebrating Levia pregnant with Kenneth

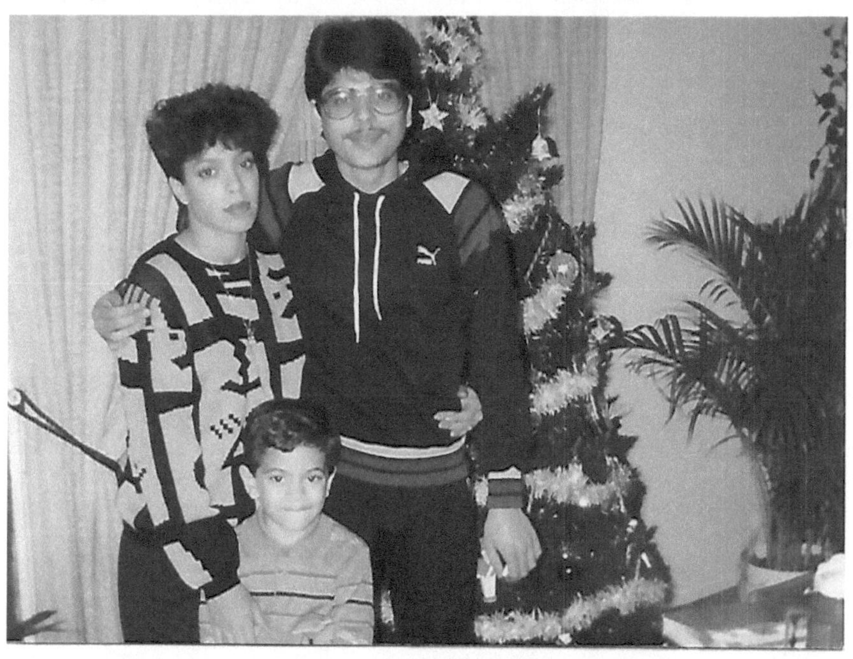

Levia Manny and Me at Christmas

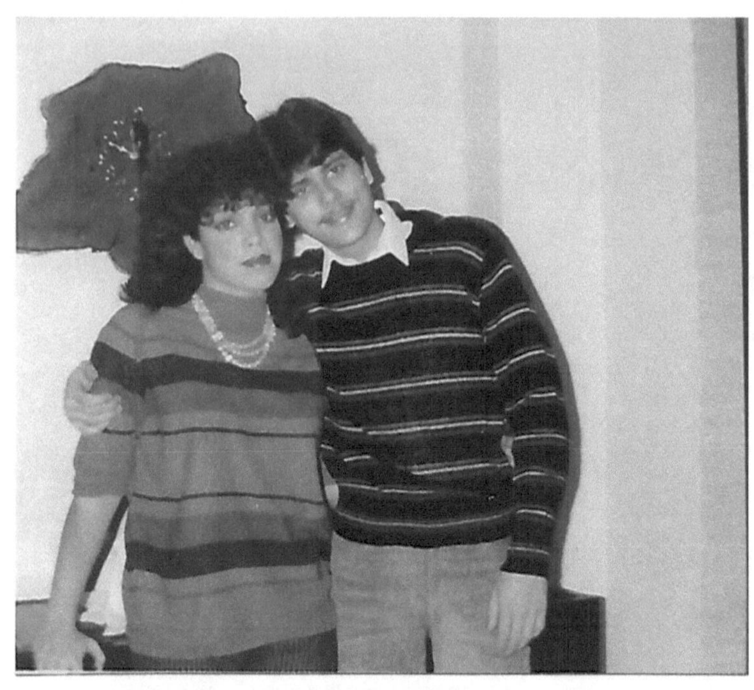

Levia and Me young

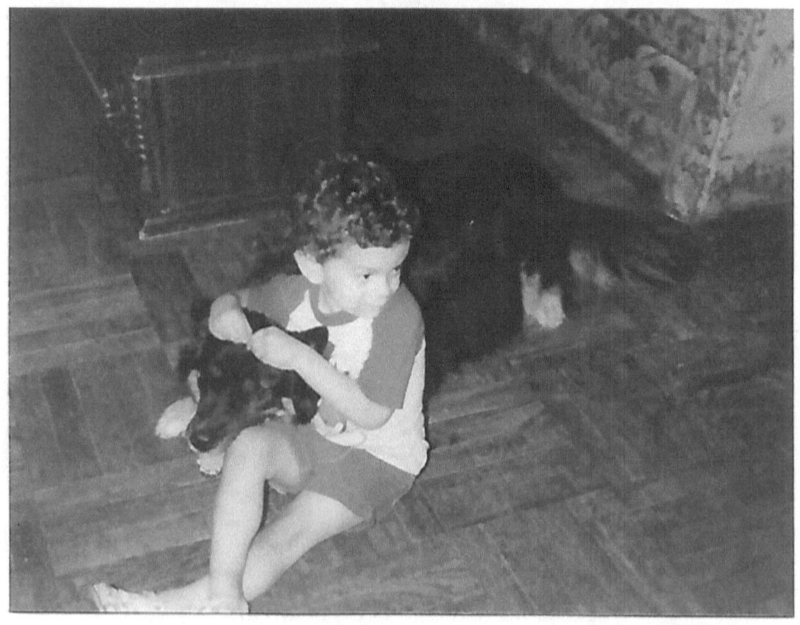

Manny with his K-9 Babysitter Candy his favorite dog

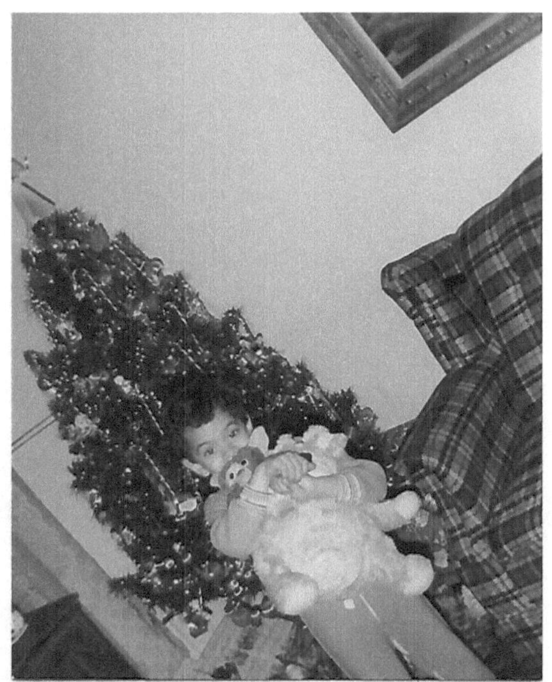

Manny and his three favorite things Christmas
Gizmo and his bunny pillow

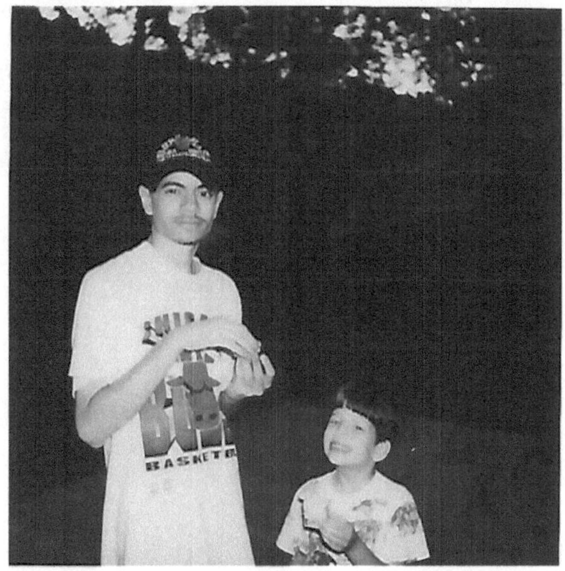

Manny and Kenneth Camping in Roscoe

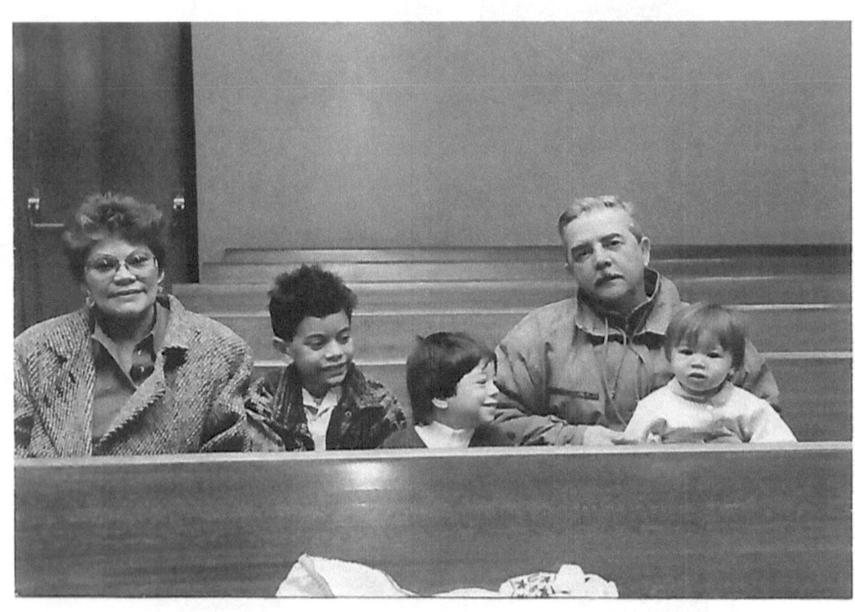

Manny with Grandma Grandpa James and Michael his cousins

# Acknowledgments

WE WOULD LIKE to thank Susan Edelman from the bottom of our hearts. Without you, Manny's story may have never been told. You started the ball rolling.

Special thanks to Christine Quinn for hearing a mother's plea and answering that plea and for proposing a law to make Manny's tragic death have meaning so that he did not die in vain. You hold a special place in our hearts, and we consider you a part of the family.

To NYS senator Thomas Duane, thanks so much for taking the bill up to Albany and making Manny's Law a state law. I know that you aren't acknowledged enough for your efforts. Therefore, we want to thank you for all that you have done for us.

To Assemblyman Pete Grannis, you are really not given the credit that is your due. So thank you so much for all your efforts and also for making Manny's law a reality.

Special thanks to our attorney, Mitch Carlinsky, for being the only one who would take the time to bring justice for Manny. Your patience and dedication and compassion made a difficult time a little more bearable.

To Dr. Sabrina Johnson, thanks so much for being the only one who cared for Manny. You stuck up for Manny when no one else would. May God bless you!

Dr. Anthony Tomasso, thanks for being the professional you are. You have taken care of us for many years now. I couldn't imagine not having you as our family doctor. Thanks for finding Kenneth's illness and being part of saving his life.

Heartfelt thanks to Dr. Gurmohan Syali. Thanks for being a man of honor with impeccable ethics. You saved our youngest son's life, and we will never forget you, ever. We consider you part of our family. May God bless you and your family forever!

Dr. Joseph Cirrone, thanks for your part in healing Kenneth and for your thoroughness and for explaining things in such a manner that we could understand.

To the entire staff at NSHOA in Patchogue, words cannot express our gratitude in the way that you cared for Kenneth. You guys are truly exceptional, and your professionalism is second to none. We thank you from the bottom of our hearts. You guys saved a life that is precious to us, and we will never forget you guys. Love you guys always. The Prieto family.

To Bay Shore High School, BOCES, and the Long Island Culinary Academy. Thanks for educating our son Manny and for giving him a respected profession.

And finally, Monica Mejia, thanks for your wonderful gift of Manny's headstone. Because of you, our son no longer has an unmarked grave. You have our love forever.